What Beth's Clients

"There is something about Beth that makes you dig deep. That makes you challenge and push yourself every day. What is even more noticeable than the physical changes are the internal changes: the confidence and the positivity. She has been so instrumental in changing my life that *Thank you* will never be enough."

—Eileen

"Over the years, Beth has continued to remind me that I can do anything I set my mind to and be whoever I want to be— something we all seem to forget over the course of our adult life. She has encouraged me to face my fears, go after my dreams, and has helped me to evolve into someone I knew I wanted to become on more levels than just fitness. And she reminds me to keep positive along the way!"

—Alisson

"Beth has not only taught me how to train and eat right but also how to push myself in a way that has actually gotten me results. Beth is not just a trainer—she is an absolute mentor. She makes you *want* to be accountable to yourself, your training, and your nutrition. She always knows how to be encouraging without being intimidating and all while helping you to achieve your goals (and then set new ones)."

—Lauren

"Amazing, inspiring, motivating, sensational, fabulous, focused, determined, supporting, caring, uplifting, awesome … I could go on and on and on about life-changer Beth Linder-Moss! She is all these things and so much more!"

—Jackie

"She has taken a girl who never exercised and showed her how to have fun *while* exercising. I have become a different person because of her."

—Anna

"Beth never gives up on you, even when you want to give up on yourself. I have had times in my journey where I've lost focus and direction. Beth never gave up on me. She encouraged me to come back and start again."

—Brienne

"I'm feeling better than I've felt in years! I could not be more *thankful* for Beth! I've never been more confident. I used to eat healthy foods but did everything else wrong. I ate the wrong portions, ate too late at night, sometimes ate too much, and other days I'd hardly eat at all. Sticking with Beth's nutrition guide, I've learned to control all of that and be on a schedule. Some days, I find that if I'm stress eating, fruit is enough natural sugar to feed that craving! *She believed she could and so she did!*"

—Val

THINK
HEALTHY
Be Healthy

Simple Strategies to Gain Confidence
Through Fitness, Nutrition,
and a Well-Balanced Lifestyle

BETH LINDER-MOSS

THINK HEALTHY, BE HEALTHY

Simple Strategies to Gain Confidence Through Fitness, Nutrition, and a Well-Balanced Lifestyle

For permission requests, speaking inquiries, and bulk order purchase options, email info@bethlinder-moss.com.

bethlinder-moss.com
Stronger Than You Think Books

ISBN-13: 979-8-218-01401-8

Library of Congress Control Number: 2019916133

Designed by Transcendent Publishing
Edited by Dragonflywings.Ink, a division of Lori Lynn Enterprises LLC
Cover Photography by Scott Roth
Initial Content Compiled by Marissa Waraksa

The content of this book is for informational purposes only and is not intended to diagnose, treat, cure, or prevent any condition or disease. You understand that this book is not intended as a substitute for consultation with a licensed practitioner. Please consult with your own physician or healthcare specialist regarding the suggestions and recommendations made in this book.

Printed in the United States of America

The best investment you can make
is in your own health.

*To my family, who have been encouraging me
to step outside my comfort zone by writing this book
and sharing my expertise with everyone.*

Contents

"The greatest wealth
is health."

—Virgil

Introduction

Susan suffered from depression for many years. She was an emotional eater who did not like to exercise. We worked together on making small, healthy changes to her diet, implementing small, manageable ways to fit in some exercise (like parking her car at the very end of the parking lot, for example), and short, five-minute meditations.

She was skeptical and nervous about even trying my approach because she'd tried so many fad diets and fitness plans before, but I invited her to simply set small, realistic weekly goals.

After the first week, she started to feel a bit better about this new lifestyle. And as the weeks went on and she started to actually see the progress, she became more confident in herself and this new, healthier, and more sustainable way to live.

Since then, Susan has been able to maintain this healthy life-style—*for years*. She has become someone who loves to work out daily, has learned how to make wise and healthy choices, has blood work within normal limits, and is happier than ever!

Another client, Zoe, was not overweight, but her blood work showed elevated cholesterol levels, her blood pressure was high, she had low bone density (a sign of osteoporosis), and she suffered from anxiety. Although her weight was within normal limits, she still needed to learn how to make healthy food choices, incorporate fitness into her daily routine, and learn some relaxation tips.

After a few months of implementing the strategies I taught her, Zoe was able to maintain normal cholesterol levels, a normal blood pressure, and has learned tips on how to deal with her anxiety.

Sometimes the stressors of everyday life make it seem like we do not have enough time or capacity to lead a healthy lifestyle. And when we feel like there are not enough minutes in the day, our willingness to motivate ourselves to work toward a healthy lifestyle starts to fade.

We either give up or we fail to spare some time for exercising, eating healthy, or meditating. Then suddenly, we find a new diet plan on the internet that we apply in an attempt to try to shed unbelievable amounts of weight within a few days. We do not consider the side effects of that diet plan because all we want is to lose weight and become healthy quickly.

Most of the time, the result is the same. Usually, you gain all the weight back once you are done with the diet because it was not a permanent fix, it was unrealistic, and it was not sustainable.

If this sounds like a relatable event to you, trust me, there are many others fighting the same battle you are. Millions of people have been there, experienced their own tipping points, and failed to understand the whole thing.

When my dad experienced his first heart attack, I was only sixteen years old. It was a tremendous shock to our family, and that's when we all started to understand the importance of a healthy lifestyle.

We each altered our diets as we moved toward a better healthy routine. That experience was what sparked my initial interest in the health/fitness field, and that is where I began my lifelong career. My father recently celebrated his eightieth birthday, and I am proud to say that he, like the rest of my family, now thinks healthy to be healthy.

You see, I wanted to write this book for a long time but could not figure out how to get started. Before I ever wrote a single word, I knew that I wanted to call it *Think Healthy, Be Healthy*. This title defines how I think about fitness, eating well, and living a balanced, positive lifestyle.

This book serves as a holistic approach to bettering your health and your happiness. You will learn how to restructure your routines to create the healthiest version of yourself. This is a complete guide that will walk you through the four components of a healthy lifestyle: Diet, Stress, Sleep, and Fitness.

I practice what I preach, and my family members have also adapted their own healthy habits as I've navigated this journey to wellness.

To get started with this book, I had to get out of my comfort zone.

I often tell my clients to push themselves, and that if they come to a point where they think they can't continue, they should just take one more step. So that is what I have done with this book—*push myself!* I did take the next step, and now, here we are … a book!

Everyone knows that they must eat right, exercise, sleep well, and de-stress throughout the day, yet most have come to believe that the hustle and bustle of everyday life make it impossible to do it all. Kids, family, furry friends, and a career get in the way.

This is the moment where I am intervening. I am going to teach you strategies and provide you with tips and tricks on how to *Think Healthy, Be Healthy.*

In this book, you will learn how you can easily balance your life by making simple, healthy changes to your diet and focusing more on your physical and mental health—all without compromising your daily life.

Being a certified Health and Wellness Coach, Personal and Group Fitness Trainer, Sports Nutritionist, and Exercise Physiologist, I am innately aware that our minds and bodies share a strong connection.

Every little change you make with your body directly affects your mind and vice versa. For example, when you are nervous, you may have used the saying, "I have butterflies in my stomach." You may be experiencing some anxiety, an emotion that activates you physiologically by causing your heart rate to rise or the feeling of butterflies swirling in your stomach. This is your mind projecting its nervousness onto your body.

Many of my past and present patients, clients, family, and friends have all seen difficult times and have developed *learned helplessness*. Going about weight loss in the wrong direction often leads to gaining the weight back, accompanied by some extra pounds. It is high time for you to break the yo-yo dieting cycle and get yourself onto a real health track.

I have been in this profession for over thirty years and I have rarely, if ever, seen any of these fad diets be truly effective with long-term success. If you genuinely wish to make yourself fit, in all aspects of that word, then you need to focus on making some essential changes to your not-so-healthy lifestyle.

Crash diets are not what you need, and you don't need to restrict your diet too much, either. All you need is a plan made for *you*. Then you must follow the plan that is most suitable for you and that serves to help you *think healthy* and therefore, *be healthy*!

I hope to share the knowledge I have attained regarding my extreme passion for health and wellness. I intend to help you develop a thought pattern that helps you to be healthy. I would like very much for you to benefit from my education, expertise, and passion. This book is a platform for me to share my enthusiasm and life experiences.

Recently, while scrolling through social media, I came across a quote that instantly grabbed my attention:

> *"Your mind is a powerful thing. When you filter it with positive thoughts, your life will start to change."*
>
> **—Gautama Buddha**

I am a firm believer in the concept that *the process of adopting a healthy lifestyle starts with developing the right mindset.* Shaping all your perspectives into a positive mold is the key ingredient to this recipe for weight loss and healthy eating.

You need to align your thoughts in the right direction. Then, take all of the negative thoughts and behaviors out of your life, and *turn them around.*

I have devoted myself to helping you learn the skills and gain the confidence you need to do what needs to be done. Before we begin this journey, I want you to first ask yourself, *Why do I need a lifestyle change? Is it to lose weight, prevent diseases, become more fit, be happier, less stressed, or have more energy?*

Once you have answered this stream of questions, you will know why you are doing this and you will have your goal in your hand—it will be clear. This clarity of knowing your goal and having a purpose is what you will need to keep yourself motivated and be prepared to start a new routine.

The vast majority of women devote their lives and efforts to everything and everyone except for themselves. They share the common view that taking time out for themselves makes them selfish. However, I want you to understand that having "me time" is not selfish! No matter how old or young you are, *you need yourself* more than anyone else does.

And on top of that, who will take care of everyone if you're too burnt out to do so?! I believe that it is extremely important for you to make time for yourself every day and to give your mind and body the necessary time to be healthy.

You can meditate, work out, go for a walk, do yoga, or listen to your favorite songs. In fact, nearly everything that makes you happy and relaxes your mind and body is your perfect therapy. A healthy mindset requires an emphasis on living a positive life.

Instead of choosing big targets to achieve, I suggest and encourage you to start by taking small steps at the beginning of this full mind-body transformation. For example, if your goal is to lose weight, start by cutting out some unhealthy eating habits and adding more physical activity.

You need to understand that how much you weigh today is not something you gained overnight. It took months or even years for you to reach this place, and similarly, the reverse mechanism is going to take some time as well.

There is no magic trick or miracle that will turn you into your ideal shape within a day or even a week. Do not expect to shed ten pounds in the blink of an eye. If you keep your expectations unrealistic, they will only let you down and make you feel like you are failing.

Refuse to fall prey to those doubts by setting healthy, realistic goals.

We would all love that magic pill—even I would. Unfortunately, it doesn't exist. Remember that it's going to take some time, but the outcome is going to be worth it. All you need is to be realistic and consistent with your goals.

Small steps serve as milestones that add up to that big achievement you work to earn through your committed practice. If you focus on the step in front of you, you will not get overwhelmed by the staircase ahead.

In the four parts of the book, I will discuss how you can lose or maintain a healthy weight and improve your mental health. First, however, I would like to give you a glance at how this is all going to work and what benefits come with this lifestyle.

I believe that nutrition is one of the most important factors to consider when it comes to maintaining a healthy lifestyle. Once the mind is aligned in the right direction, all the magic lies in the kitchen. As they say, "Abs are made in the kitchen!"

You must have a diet that provides your body with the necessary nutrients, and make sure that whatever food you consume is healthy and free from excessive sugars and carbs. The secret to good nutrition lies in the idea of balancing your proteins, carbohydrates, fruits, fats, vegetables, and water intake.

I will help you understand the differences between the good and bad subcategories that exist within each of these food groups. Then, I will guide you accordingly in how to cut down or eliminate unhealthy foods from your diet while refocusing on the healthier options.

Physical health has a lot to do with the physical activities that a person keeps themselves busy with, as well. Of course, this isn't earth-shattering news. Food will treat some of your health concerns, but activity is equally important.

Your physical activity plays a vital role in improving your physical and mental health. A good workout helps you burn calories and increases the serotonin levels in your body, making you happier and more relaxed.

Regular exercise can turn out to be extremely beneficial for you, and you will feel the benefits in just a few days. There are numerous health benefits to having a regular workout and so many ways to get it in, as you will see in the upcoming chapters.

Exercise does not necessarily have to be a set of crunches or a round of push-ups. It can be as simple as taking your dog for walks, yoga, hiking, biking, swimming, group fitness classes, paddleboarding, or even walking to a friend's house around the block.

I take great pride in saying openly that I have successfully implemented these lifestyle changes within my own family. I have always instilled a necessary balance between my family members' healthy diet and physical activity.

My kids enjoy eating the typical kiddie foods most kids eat—just in healthy moderation. I do not believe in restricting or cutting off anything from diets, rather, limiting it to the right amount. You should be able to eat everything you like, but just make sure you eat it in moderation and exercise regularly.

In the end, it is all about the right balance of food and exercise.

My favorite aspect of having a healthy body is the energized feeling you obtain. Lethargy is a common feeling many people exhibit. They just don't have the energy to perform their daily chores over time. And over the years, I've come across so many clients who would complain constantly about having low energy levels.

Most of them would tell me about the crazy diets they had tried. They'd also mention that they would go for sporadic exercise and other remedies to make themselves feel better again, but of course, I always tell them that all they need is a healthy balance between nutrition and fitness.

I believe in living the healthiest and happiest life possible. Through my journey, I have had the distinct pleasure of helping countless people discover the way to lead a healthy lifestyle—a healthy lifestyle they can sustain.

In the upcoming chapters, you will learn how a balanced diet, regular physical activity, and a good sleep routine can greatly reduce your stress levels and lead you toward a happier and more active life. You will also learn about the astonishing effects of fitness, food choices, yoga, and mediation, among other strategies to help you lead a happy and healthy lifestyle.

And on top of it all, you will learn how to implement these methodologies in a way that is easy to incorporate into your life to start paving the way for change *now*.

 The main purpose of this book is to inspire you to live a healthy, fun, energetic life. Living this kind of lifestyle can help you to prevent chronic illnesses, such as heart disease, diabetes, high blood pressure, obesity, back pain, strokes, osteoporosis, depression, and cholesterol issues.

 Living a truly healthy lifestyle can teach you how to manage any pre-existing conditions that you may have. Leading a healthy life can also help to reduce the need for both prescription and over-the-counter medications and decrease overall stress levels.

More than anything, though, having a healthy body will lead to a sound mind as the healthy changes lead you to an improved mental state and help you in boosting your self-esteem and confidence.

I want you to know that *you are worth it*. You can do anything your mind is devoted to. Leading a healthy lifestyle is not as challenging as most have grown to expect. I want you to know that I am and will be by your side for your journey! I am so excited that we can do this together!

"There's nothing more important
than our good health –
That's our principal capital asset."

—Arlen Specter

Who Is Beth Linder-Moss?

*I*n high school, I was a gymnast—not a very good one, but I was on the varsity team. I only lettered because I was on the team for all four years of high school. Unlike today's typical gymnast who practices four hours a day, I didn't spend so many long hours on it. Nutrition and fitness didn't have a place in my life the way they do now, however, being a gymnast was a lifesaver for me because it helped me maintain being in good shape.

Then, when I was a senior in high school and gymnastics was over, I joined an all-women's gym with my sister. I loved taking aerobic classes. They made me feel good, and I had so much fun while staying in shape.

Sometimes I feel like I should be paying credit to those classes for how they helped to steer me into the fitness/health world. Even after thirty years, I still love fitness classes—whether I am teaching them or one of the participants. I love how they make me feel, and I cherish seeing how it makes other people feel about themselves.

I've been lucky enough to have helped encourage and motivate thousands of people to change their lives for the better. I have gained so much knowledge through both my continued education and by simply *living what I teach.*

My passion for sharing my knowledge to benefit others through education is intense and is forever pushing me a step further, past my limits. I look forward to leaving a positive impression on as many peoples' lives as possible through both my personal and professional experiences.

I believe the key to a healthy lifestyle is moderation because an excess of anything could harm you. In my home, I have set norms and values that my kids and husband follow on a regular basis to live a healthy and balanced life. Since my kids were toddlers, I have been informing them about the benefits of eating healthy and exercising.

I don't believe in overdoing any aspect of a healthy lifestyle. I believe in maintaining a healthy and manageable balance. Therefore, my children have learned the good and bad aspects of a healthy lifestyle, and as such, I do not need to restrict or guide them anymore. For example, if they have a cupcake or ice cream at a friend's birthday party, they know that they should not have any more sweets later that day.

I cannot stress enough the importance of moderation. You need to make sure that you are enjoying the foods that bring you pleasure while also maintaining a balance of intake. I don't recall ever stopping my children from having chocolates or any other junk food unless they had had it already, earlier in the day.

If you completely cut the items you love out of your diet, you will most likely binge. You might be tempted to eat those foods in excess when you go out because you are craving them or missing them. When craving these items, you are more likely to cheat on your diet.

The trends are too high to ignore *because they're true!* That is why it is not recommended to cut off any foods completely, but rather, to have them in moderation along with the other healthy foods you consume.

I always ensure my pantry has all the foods that my kids love. I keep chocolates, ice cream, marshmallows, and other unhealthy snacks for them. By doing so, I make sure they don't feel like they are missing out on these delightful snacks. They need to satisfy their taste buds by enjoying the snack in moderation. If these snacks were completely off-limits for them, they would go out and munch on their favorites in larger—and thus, unhealthier—quantities.

I always tell my family, friends, and clients, "You need to be healthy in order to take care of your loved ones." If you are not physically and mentally well, then how can you expect to help others?

Take the example of being on an airplane. I think that it fits accurately into the scenario of maintaining a state of wellness. The infamous announcement comes on: In case of an emergency, the oxygen mask will automatically drop down. Make sure you put yours on first before helping the other people around you.

I am a proud mother of a twenty-year-old son and two beautiful sixteen-year-old twin daughters. I love how they trust and follow me in carrying out a healthy lifestyle. They truly understand the importance of physical and mental well-being. It is a cornerstone I raised them with!

Throughout their childhood, I have told them that, as their mother, I need to be healthy in order to care for them. I feel this really helped them to understand why I had to take time out of each day to work out. I also feel they benefited from seeing a healthy lifestyle modeled for them.

Now that they are teenagers, I love working out with them. We all go on hikes, bike rides, paddleboard trips, or kayak trips, go swimming at the beach or to yoga sessions, and go on runs together. My son loves to go rock-climbing and surf for hours, and my girls will play soccer and field hockey, or surf for hours on end, as well. I encourage them to do it all!

Everyone should take the chance to start enjoying fun and mind-refreshing activities with their families. Leading by example is key, and when you can have fun doing it all together, it makes it all the better! You may not even feel like you have to "work out" at all when you implement active family time into your routine.

It is no surprise that children will want to eat junk food or fast food, but it is important for you to know what is in the food they're eating. Most fast-food restaurants do not offer healthy options. You need to teach your children from a very young age to be healthy by choosing healthy foods and emphasizing the importance of living a healthy lifestyle.

Again, if they see *you* munching on chocolate all day long while you tell them to eat their broccoli, they may not follow through in the long run. The best impact will be made when the balanced, healthy lifestyle is modeled before their very eyes. Trust me, one day you will be so proud to see your child following the same healthy routine as you, it will make it all the more worthwhile.

When I call my son in college and he talks about the healthy food choices he makes, my heart soars. I'm so proud of him for eating well at college, knowing that he has so many other choices in front of him.

My friends have always joked about having to keep fresh fruits and vegetables around when my kids come over because that's what they ask for when having a snack. I believe the best thing we can do is teach our children how to motivate themselves to live healthier and happier lives, so we lead by example.

There is a famous quote by Asa Don Brown, "Children are sponges, soaking up every verbal and nonverbal interaction," and I couldn't agree more. Children follow the practices and routines that we set in the home, and most importantly, whatever we model before them.

My kids have been packing their own lunch boxes and snacks since they were in pre-school. I taught them how to pack them, and how to pack healthy. I taught them to add protein, fruits, vegetables, and carbohydrates to their lunch to enjoy a balanced meal.

They would pack a yogurt, apple, carrots, and pretzels or some combo such as this, all by themselves. Now, I don't need to stress over what they're eating or drinking because I'm confident they know how to decide for themselves, and I can count on their healthy choices most of the time.

Consistency and routine are the most important ingredients to a recipe for success. Even though we have thousands of reasons not to go to the gym, or to grab that quick, unhealthy snack, you can also find at least one good reason why you should make a healthier choice. And when you do, making this decision will make you feel so good and proud of yourself.

No matter how busy you are, you need to manage your time accordingly and be able to find the "me time" that is so needed every day. There will be days when you will be caught up by many things, with so much on your plate that you won't have time for long exercise sessions, and that is fine.

Sometimes, my children are so occupied with their schoolwork or assignments that they cannot fit in a 30–minute workout session. So instead, they make it a point to get in 10–15 minutes of physical activity, as they know full well how important it is and how good it makes them feel.

I am sharing some of my health routines with you because I want to inspire you to implement the same values and routines in your homes. I think women in particular need to be conscious of how they take care of themselves.

By this, I do not mean in any way that a man's health is less important, but I do believe that a woman's body goes through a lot of changes. Therefore, we need to take care of every little thing that's going on in our bodies.

For example, when I was pregnant, exercise and yoga immensely helped me to enjoy a safe pregnancy. They also helped me get back into shape quickly after delivery. Even when pregnant with my twins, my doctor allowed me to take daily walks and do soothing yoga sessions to feel good. It did wonders for my body and mind.

I was not allowed to do any type of vigorous workouts during pregnancy, but I was able to enjoy all the other physical activities I wanted to do during that time. If your body is already used to these fitness activities, then it gets easier for you to continue them throughout your pregnancy.

I want you to know that physical and mental fitness is not a luxury, *it is a necessity*. Your overall activities and exercises, from cardio, strength training, yoga, and meditation to enjoying a balanced diet, should be a constant part of your life.

For example, you brush your teeth every morning after you wake up, or perhaps you have a cup of hot coffee right after you shower each morning. So why not treat your physical and mental exercises the same way? Make them an integral part of your routine.

If you can do these physical and mental activities with friends, it could be a time where you socialize. You might make a few new friends at the gym, too. And when you have workout buddies, they can help to hold you accountable. In fact, you can hold each other accountable. It helps when you have a strong core group or a friend who is on the same health journey as you!

How many times a week do you wake up in the morning feeling lethargic or cranky? Despite getting seven or eight hours of peaceful sleep, you feel as though you were up all night. There's a reason behind this—you may not be moving your body enough! Believe it or not, studies show that a large percentage of health problems exist because people remain stuck in one place all day long.

Hey, maybe you just don't feel like getting up from your couch, bed, or office chair. Most of us work in an office or someplace where we remain seated for eight to ten hours a day. You're by no means alone in experiencing this limitation on consistent physical movement.

If this is you, then before you relax or do anything else, take thirty to forty minutes when you get home at the end of the day to work out. Try taking a few five-minute walking breaks around the office or your home. If you're a morning person, you could implement your physical workout routine first thing in the morning. You can do exercises at home, hit the gym, or even just go for a walk during your lunch break.

You will quickly see amazing benefits for your body and mind. Exercise can help to eliminate brain fog, enhance mental clarity, and promote higher levels of concentration. Once you start your exercise routine, you will feel the difference in your energy levels. Instead of needing that second cup of coffee, you will wake up feeling energized and ready to take on the day.

If you have successfully implemented new ideas and traditions in your family, then why not pass them on to future generations, as well? In the same way I guide my family by example, you can also demonstrate to your children how to implement this idea of a healthy lifestyle so that the following generations also benefit from them, leaving a legacy of wellness behind you.

Recently, I came across a very meaningful quote by Josh Billings that states, "Health is like money. We never have a true idea of its value until we lose it." I find this quote to be accurate and relatable to my experience with my father's heart attack when I was a teenager.

Health is indeed like money. People never realize the true value of their health unless they are faced with an acute chronic disease or a disorder. We need to take care of our health so we can try to avoid any diseases or chronic illnesses.

I exercise every day and eat a very healthy diet, but my fitness routine isn't boring. I still have a wide variety of options for healthy eating and exercising. I mix up my daily workouts with HIIT (High-Intensity Interval Training), yoga, strength, and outdoor activities like paddleboarding, hiking, and long walks with my dog.

I want all of you to know that I absolutely practice what I preach. And as you get to know me, you will see this as true. Trust me when I say that you will not want to turn back once you embark on this journey of wellness. You will love all the energy and health benefits that come with it.

As you follow your new schedule with daily exercise and healthy eating, you will see that it is not hard to stick with. I will not lie, it may take a few weeks to get into a routine, but this schedule will quickly turn into a habit!

PART ONE
Lifestyle

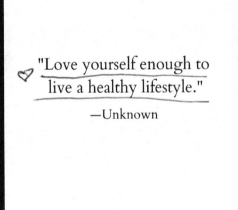

"Love yourself enough to
live a healthy lifestyle."

—Unknown

Building a Healthy Foundation

*E*very woman wants to be healthy, which is easier said than done. In our busy lives, we feel that maintaining a healthy lifestyle requires a lot of time and effort. We have so much on our plates, and we tend to think that adding the task of "staying healthy" to it all is only going to make things more difficult. Even now, some of you may be overwhelmed by the sheer idea of trying to be healthy, getting fit, or being more active.

Whenever we find some time to work on our healthy habits, we tend to overcomplicate it, thinking we need to do more, restrict more, count more, and push our bodies past their limits. On the contrary, it does not have to be complicated, does not take much time, and the benefits you gain are far beyond the efforts required.

Our busy and overachieving minds compartmentalize health as something to be done in addition to the hundred other things on our to-do lists. But health and wellness should not be another thing that demands more from us, instead, they should be seamlessly woven into our daily lives in a way that serves *us* well and supports all aspects of *our* physical and mental health.

Sounds good, right? However, we all know that it is not a walk in the park (though it literally should be).

Maintaining a healthy lifestyle is a slow process, as you will need to incorporate small changes into your life over time, but it's also less complicated than you may think. Today's women underestimate the effects that small, incremental habit changes can have on us.

We think that we will be healthier if we follow crash diets, take on extreme workouts, or perform heavy weightlifting, but that is simply not the case. **The foundation of your healthy lifestyle is based on the formation of small habits that you incorporate into your daily life.**

Building a healthy foundation and getting into a healthy lifestyle is as easy as engaging in small movements throughout the day to keep yourself active and energized. For example, climbing the stairs instead of taking the elevator, walking over to a co-worker instead of emailing them, or going for a ten-minute walk midday.

These small movements will improve your blood circulation, metabolism, digestion, and energy levels. Moreover, movement will also have a huge impact on your mental health. You will feel a noticeable decline in your stress levels, mood tantrums, and general grumpiness.

I am proposing that you implement small changes into your routine. But how do you make sure these small changes stick?

For example, if you learned that there were benefits to taking a fish oil supplement daily, how would you make sure to take it regularly? You would need to form a habit. Doing something every day for twenty-one days in a row turns it into a new habit, no matter what it is. If you want to enjoy the health benefits of fish oil, then you would need to take fish oil every day for at least twenty-one days.

After that time, your mind and body would've had enough time to accept this change into your routine. In the initial days of taking fish oil supplements, you might have forgotten to take it one or two days in a row, as you had not developed the habit yet. Eventually, after twenty-one days, you get used to your new habit, and from that point on, you will be able to stick to it for as long as you want.

Your healthy habits can become part of your life if you remain consistent in following through with them. Some of you may be thinking that twenty-one days is too much time. It really isn't though—it's only three weeks. And how much of your life is three weeks, really?

I have come up with some tips and techniques that can help you to slowly start building your own solid foundation of healthy practices. Your healthy habits *will* result in more health, wellness, and overall happiness.

"The secret of your
future is hidden
in your daily routine."

—Mike Murdock

How to Create Healthy Habits

*F*irst, you need to focus on what new habit you want to implement in your life. For example, let's say you want to get into the habit of doing a thirty-minute workout session every day. The first thing you need to do is set a time frame dedicated to your physical workout. You can pick any time slot that works for you. One important thing here is that it isn't necessary for you to stick to the same workout time every day.

If your work shifts are different each day, then you can easily adjust your exercise schedule accordingly. For example, if you get back from work around 7:00 p.m. on Mondays and Tuesdays, you can exercise at 7:30 or 8:00 p.m. or even before you leave for work in the morning. Similarly, if you work night shifts the other days, you can choose mornings for your exercise routine, like 9:00 or 10:00 a.m.

Your workout schedule must work for you. If it does not, you will have a hard time sticking to it.

Although research shows that new habits can be developed within twenty-one days, I would still recommend that you commit to each new habit for at least thirty days. Some people take a little longer than others to adjust, so it is best to be sure that the habit has become part of your day-to-day life before taking a day away from it.

Again, the key is to focus on each small step instead of the big staircase in front of you. Don't focus on the twenty-one or thirty days. Mark your calendar and let it go. Then adjust your focus to the day at hand.

Take it one step at a time, and eventually, you will climb up the ladder of having a healthy lifestyle. Little adjustments will not leave you feeling overwhelmed. For example, after you drop the kids at school, try to go straight to the gym or yoga class. Or, when you get dressed in the morning, put on your workout clothes, so you are ready for your walk.

With these small changes, it will be easier for you to incorporate exercise into your routine. You'll barely notice your new pattern shift. And once these adjustments become a part of your routine, you will have developed the habit, and you will then stick with it.

Taking small steps will also motivate you to remain consistent with your health journey, which is very important. You need to stick to your health practices and routines for better results. For example, your habits might be walking ten to fifteen minutes each day, adding veggies to dinner, or getting to sleep by 10:00 p.m.

I have some clients who complain that they do not see the results they were hoping for, even after following a specific diet or exercise routine for a month. I always have one question for them: Are you consistent with your practices?

While following our health journey, we need to remember that change will not come overnight. It is going to take some time. We need to be consistent with our habits.

Your diet and exercise will not benefit you unless you practice consistency. If you eat healthy five days a week but binge on five scoops of ice cream and make unhealthy choices each weekend, then it will be hard to make progress.

Balance is extremely essential. You can eat everything so long as it's in moderation. And if your goal is to lose or maintain your weight, just watch your calorie intake as you eat.

Apart from your physical health, you need to focus on your mental health, as well. Try to stay away from stressful news, toxic people, and depressive TV shows. Choose to be as happy as you can.

Focus more on your wins! Even the smallest wins should be celebrated. For example, you can get a jar and put a dollar in it for each small win. At the end of the month, you could buy yourself a new workout shirt, take yourself out on a date or to a movie, or do something else that will motivate you to continue along your path.

Plan for days that may have obstacles, and be prepared with a backup plan for days when time and weather are not on your side. If you normally like to go for a walk every day but it's going to rain, then plan on doing mall walking or Pilates that day. This way, you will remain consistent with your habits and stay on track.

You should also track your accountability. Maintain a journal in which you note all the details of your daily food intake and fitness routine, or have an accountability partner by your side who is going on your journey with you. This will give you additional support. Plus, you will likely get more ideas from your accountability partner that you can implement on your own health journey—for example, new recipes, workouts, or yoga tutorials.

Yesterday, I came across a very meaningful quote by Dr. Wayne W. Dyer, stating, "Healthy habits are learned in the same way as unhealthy ones—through practice." Frankly, I couldn't agree more.

It's true that all types of habits take the same amount of time to form. For instance, if you ask a chain smoker how they got into the habit of smoking, they will tell you, "With time." You see, even unhealthy habits take time to become a part of our lives. Therefore, you can never expect to get used to your healthy practices overnight.

"We first make our habits,
and then
our habits make us."

—Unknown

Tips for Building
a Healthier Lifestyle

*P*hysical fitness is not the only criteria for being labeled as healthy. It is also doing well in areas of your physical and mental well-being. A healthy lifestyle can help you prevent chronic diseases, stress, anxiety, psychological disorders, and long-term illnesses. It can also help you to feel good about yourself from the inside, boosting your confidence levels and improving your focus.

Although there are numerous ways in which you can take care of your overall physical and mental well-being, I am highlighting some of the important ones in this section.

- Maintain a healthy and balanced diet (rich in protein, carbs, healthy fats, fruits, vegetables, vitamins, and fiber). Try to include more protein in each meal, it helps to boost your energy levels and metabolism. In turn, this results in weight loss and stabilized blood sugar levels.

- Exercise regularly–at least thirty to forty minutes, five days a week.

- Avoid drugs and consume alcohol in moderation, as these things could harm your physical and mental health in several ways. For instance, excess alcohol consumption could lead to diabetes, depression, anxiety, kidney failure, cardiovascular diseases, or cancer.

- Stay hydrated and make sure you drink enough water every day. Consume half of your body weight in ounces of water. Try not to exceed one hundred ounces.

- Get seven hours of sleep every night to boost your immunity and energy levels.

- Pre-plan your meals and snacks so you don't grab the unhealthy options when you are in a hurry.

- Do not skip breakfast or other meals, as it can slow your metabolism down.

- Eat a lot of vegetables and fruits to add plenty of vitamins, minerals, and fiber to your diet.

- Maintain a food and fitness log to record what you eat and what you've done for exercise each day. Be sure to mention the duration and type of physical activity in your log.

- Challenge yourself and keep growing. Do not be afraid of the little obstacles that come your way. Even on your worst days, do not forget to exercise and eat healthy. This will help you to be consistent with your health journey.

- Incorporate all types of fitness, strength, flexibility, and cardio exercises into your routine.

- Take some time out for a little relaxation each day, such as a bath, deep breathing, or meditation.

- The last but most important point is to have fun. Do not forget to occasionally treat yourself to a light cheat meal or go out with friends for a good movie. It will help you stay true to your goals.

While some of these steps may seem super simple and others extremely difficult for you, the key here is to start implementing some of them into your everyday life. Sadly, most people nowadays opt for quick fixes that are often unsustainable or unhealthy overall.

It is hard for us to embrace a slow and simple strategy in this extraordinarily advanced and modern world. But I can assure you that it is the best way to look and feel great while optimizing your health benefits. It is also the most sustainable way to maintain a healthy lifestyle.

The only rule here is to take one step at a time. No matter how many times you fail, just keep trying until you succeed. Richelle E. Goodrich says it so perfectly:

"My goals may seem impossibly far-fetched when really they're not. Break them down into steps and see how I accomplish great things. I can easily reach from A to B. I can manage from B to C. I can make it from C to D. And so eventually, I will find my way from A to Z."

Despite being small, these changes truly have the power to transform your life and change it for the better.

"Every human being
is the author of his own
health or disease."

—Swami Sivananda

Living a Healthy Lifestyle

*W*e tell ourselves that we are doing everything possible to be happy, live healthy, and build the best lives for ourselves and our families. Do you really believe that what you're telling yourself is true?

Are you living a healthy life that makes you stronger every day? Most of us think we do. Apart from occasionally getting off track over the weekends or by binging on fudgy brownies during movie nights, you believe you are leading a perfectly healthy lifestyle for the rest of the week.

According to a recent study published in *The Archives of Internal Medicine*, very few adults in the United States meet the four criteria for a healthy lifestyle. The study showed that only 3% of Americans got a perfect score on what the authors define as a healthy life. Moreover, only 13.8% met three of the criteria, and 34.2% met only two points from the criteria.

Crazy, right?! However, the same study showed that women scored slightly better than men.

According to the abovementioned study, the four criteria of a healthy lifestyle are **a balanced diet, low stress, the correct amount of sleep, and consistent exercise**. Now ask yourself the question from earlier, but a bit differently: Do my family and I meet the four criteria? Or at least three?

In this section of the book, I intend to successfully walk you down this road of living a healthy lifestyle while teaching you which factors contribute to making our lives healthier. Although there are several ways in which you can live a physically and mentally healthy life, I will be specifically highlighting the ones I have found to be the most impactful.

You can truly enjoy a healthy and happy life if you take care of these four criteria because just about every other aspect of a healthy lifestyle falls under these categories in one way or another. But this raises the question: How can we take care of these things every single day?

Improving your health could be as easy as switching from white pasta to chickpea or lentil pasta, adding a tablespoon of chia seeds to your regular oatmeal bowl, or making your coffee with skim or almond milk instead of whole milk.

To improve your health, you might need to take daily walks, stretch, and meditate several times a week or adjust your eating habits. Making little changes to your diet and adding physical fitness can result in big health benefits.

A good mental state can only be achieved when you create the right headspace by replacing all your negative thoughts with a better perspective and by sleeping well. Sleeping well is something one must really commit to if it's going to make the necessary difference. We must allow ourselves to get an adequate amount of sleep at night—nothing over or under the specified number of hours is considered "sleeping well."

PART TWO

Diet

"Your life does not
get better with chance.
It gets better with change."

—Jim Rohn

What Is a Healthy Diet?

Your physical and mental wellbeing is directly related to what you eat and drink. The nutrients your body craves can all be obtained through what you eat. All these nutrients and minerals will help you excel throughout the day.

A balanced diet consists of fruits, vegetables, proteins, fats, and whole grains (carbohydrates). In order to stay healthy, you need to make sure that your intake of fluids, macronutrients, micronutrients, and calories is sufficient every day.

You should be aware of the different types of fats, carbs, nutrients, and proteins. Accordingly, you must be able to differentiate these foods. Your diet should be low in saturated fats, trans fats, and excessive cholesterol.

Foods high in cholesterol or trans fats may cause your body to develop chronic health problems such as diabetes, obesity, or cardiovascular disease. Some foods to eat once in a while or to avoid eating entirely are fried foods, cheese, butter, fatty meats, cookies, and cakes.

Apart from these, a healthy diet is also low in sugar and salt. Excess sugar and salt can lead to water retention, bloating, inflammation in the body, diabetes, high blood pressure, and obesity.

Sticking to a healthy diet isn't as difficult as it seems because all you need to do is replace your regular oily, fatty meals with healthy ones. For example, you can use sweet potato instead of white potato, as it will not spike your body's insulin levels. Or you can use brown rice instead of white rice to avoid obesity or diabetes-related complications.

Similarly, you can add stevia (it's made from a leaf) to your coffees, smoothies, or desserts rather than sugar. Or you can switch to honey to manage your blood sugar levels.

As we talk about healthier food choices, we have many options. Even the slightest amount of change in your eating habits will benefit your body and make you fit and healthy again. Remember, you were fit and healthy at one point in time, and the goal is to reclaim that feeling.

When you are snacking, replace your mayonnaise dips with mustard, avocado, or salsa. Trust me, these changes will be close to your heart once they're adopted. You will feel lighter and less bloated. You will feel *better*.

Even when making your veggie plate, you can replace iceberg lettuce with romaine to get more nutrients and minerals. The

USDA provides the following nutrition information for one cup of romaine vs iceberg lettuce:

Nutrients	Romain	Iceberg
Calories	8	8
Protein	.58 grams	.5 grams
Fiber	1 gram	.7 grams
Calcium	16 mg	.7 grams
Potassium	116 mg	78 mg
Vitamin C	11.3 mg	1.5 mg
Vitamin K	48.2 mcg	13.3 mcg
Beta carotene	163 mcg	164 mcg

Apart from romaine, there's a long list of other vegetables that are extremely beneficial for your health, including (but not limited to) cucumbers, green beans, spinach, beets, lemons, cabbage, and kale.

Many times, we prefer eating our food when it's fried, like chicken, veggies, or french fries. How about grilling, baking, broiling, or air-frying them instead? It will help you to enjoy healthier meals without unhealthy oils and with less fats involved.

Seeds and nuts play an integral part in maintaining a well-balanced, healthy diet. Make sure that you are including plenty of fiber-rich seeds in your daily meals, yogurt, and smoothies.

Fiber is something that should be included because it helps to cleanse your body. For example, adding chia, sunflower, flax, or pumpkin seeds can be a great source for adding extra fiber and omega-3 fatty acids to your meals.

You can also add any type of nuts to your meals, like almonds, cashews, pistachios, walnuts, or pecans. Peanuts are a great choice because they are heart-healthy and have several nutrients in them, like vitamin E, niacin, folate, and protein.

Be careful which kinds of peanuts you choose because there are so many different types to eat. The best are the ones without anything added. The roasted, salted, and honey roasted all have added calories and fat.

Oftentimes, people overlook the liquids they drink when counting their consumed calories. Your hot and cold beverages add up in your daily calorie intake and are equally responsible for your health. The calories from these drinks can result in unwanted weight gain which can lead to high blood pressure or diabetes.

There are many ways in which you can enjoy healthy and delicious beverages. All you need to do is replace your regular sodas or diet sodas with flavored seltzer or water infused with fruits, both of which have no chemicals.

Water and seltzer will help your body feel less bloated, more hydrated, and will allow you to cut back on the unnecessary calories. You can also replace your ice-cream smoothies with regular fruit smoothies. Moreover, you can use almond milk, coconut milk, or skim milk in your coffee, smoothies, or oatmeal.

Substituting 2/3 cup of skim milk in your oats instead of water can add:

- 6 grams of quality protein
- 255 mg of potassium
- 205 mg calcium
- 14% of the recommended dietary intake for vitamin B-12
- 67 IU of vitamin D

Sounds amazing, doesn't it? And these are just some of the healthy diet changes you can easily apply and incorporate into your everyday meals, snacks, and beverages.

You know that protein is one of your best friends because it keeps you full longer, helps in building muscles, helps to stabilize blood sugars, plays a role in hormone regulation, and aids in weight loss. Therefore, you should incorporate lean protein sources into your diet like chicken, tofu, eggs, turkey, yogurt, fish, cottage cheese, or plant-based protein options.

In the "How to Create Healthy Habits" section of this book, I mention keeping a journal. Another great way to keep track of your diet is by maintaining a food diary or keeping a food journal to record whatever you eat throughout the day and hold yourself accountable. The major purpose of keeping this record is to see what you consume for meals and snacks and to keep track of your water and beverage intake throughout the day.

Suppose you had a fruit smoothie with chia seeds and coffee with almond milk for breakfast. In your food log, you would write down how much fruit you added, how many tablespoons of chia seeds, how much coffee, and how much almond milk you added. And you would continue to do this with everything you eat and drink throughout the day.

Each day's record is maintained in this diary and then analyzed at the end of the week to see the progress you have made. This weekly progress report will not only allow you to see what you have been eating, but it will also boost your motivation and willingness for continuing to adopt such minor changes to bring out major differences.

I personally always forget what I ate earlier in the morning by the time dinner comes around. I also believe that I will not grab an extra handful of pretzels or any other snacks as I walk through my kitchen because I do not want them to be on my food diary.

So throughout the day, as you add your solids and liquids to your food diary, keep in mind that you are holding yourself accountable so that:

1. You do not forget *what and how much* you ate.

2. You avoid eating things you know you do not need in your diet—especially because if you eat it, you will have to write it down and then look at it at the end of the week.

All in all, we can conclude that we need to keep away from processed foods, excessive carbs, and oily and sugary foods. Instead, we must learn to enjoy whole and unprocessed foods—they are the delicacies that are best for your physical and mental health.

Remember, I am not asking you to completely cut out everything else from your diet. As discussed earlier, you can enjoy everything in moderation.

Most of your diet should consist of fruits, vegetables, whole grains, healthy fats, protein sources, and fiber. However, once you make these adjustments and substitutions, you will feel the magic of eating healthy.

"A healthy outside starts
from the inside."

—Robert Urich

Healthy Eating

*W*hether you are re-evaluating your eating habits to fit into your favorite clothes or to reach new health goals, it is never a bad time to be more thoughtful about the fuel you are putting into your body. Balanced eating is the cornerstone of good health. Like men, women should also enjoy a nutrient-rich diet consisting of all the food groups, including whole grains, fruits, vegetables, healthy fats, low-fat dairy, and lean protein.

According to research, women need to be more specific about their diet than men because their bodies go through more physical and hormonal changes as they grow older, and they also tend to have lower metabolic rates. When females hit puberty, they start developing extra nutritional requirements. Therefore, they must maintain a healthy and balanced diet starting at a young age.

It is a fact that women need fewer calories than men, but our requirements for certain vitamins and minerals are much higher. Due to several hormonal changes associated with menstruation, childbearing, and menopause, women are at a higher risk of developing anemia, osteoporosis, and deficiencies in calcium, magnesium, and vitamins.

Most women think that eating healthy means dieting, which is not true. Your target weight can be achieved by following a crash diet, but those diets almost never provide your body with all the essential nutrients it needs. Most women look for that one magic pill that can help them lose weight overnight.

As I have mentioned before, moderation is the key! In this section, I am going to discuss in detail how you can maintain a healthy weight (or even lose weight) by following a balanced diet.

Most of the time, you lose weight quickly if you follow extreme fad diets, but as soon as you go back to eating normally, you gain all the weight back within a few weeks or months. To lose weight, it really is calories in vs calories out.

You need to burn more calories than you consume. This is how weight loss works. However, you need to do it in a healthy way, which is a little more complex than just eating fewer calories and working out more.

As discussed in the previous section, the best way to stay healthy and maintain a healthy weight is to eat well, exercise regularly, maintain low stress levels, and create a proper sleep routine. One of the most amazing advantages of eating healthy is that it will help you to reduce the stress levels in your body, leading to better mental health. Eating healthy will also help you sleep better, giving you the ability to develop a consistent sleep routine.

Wikipedia defines healthy *eating* as eating that helps maintain or improve overall health. It provides the body with essential nutrition, fluids, macronutrients, micronutrients, and adequate calories. A healthy *diet* should include protein (animal or plant-based), carbohydrates, fruits, vegetables, low sugar, nothing processed, and healthy fats.

Healthy eating is not magic that is going to benefit you overnight. Therefore, you need to remain consistent with it.

In this part of the book, I want to look a little deeper into your body's nutritional needs. Healthy eating is all about striking the right balance between your macro and micronutrients. As you read on, I will explain more about them.

"Nutrition isn't just about eating, it's about learning to live."

—Patricia Compton

What Are Macronutrients?

You may have heard the term "macro" at some point during your weight-loss journey. Maybe you've heard people talk about calculating their macros every day to lose weight. Basically, **macronutrients are the substances that you need in larger amounts to provide nourishment for your body to function properly**, as the word "macro" means large.

Macronutrients mainly provide your body with the energy required to perform daily tasks and workouts. They are measured in the form of calories or kcal.

There are three components to macronutrients: carbohydrates, fats, and proteins.

Carbohydrates make up the biggest component of your macros. Sugar, starches, and fiber are all considered carbohydrates, or carbs, which are essential for your survival. Carbs are needed by your brain, muscles, and cells to function efficiently.

The best carbohydrates are the ones that have a slower absorption rate. They are called complex carbohydrates or complex carbs. Some complex carbs are vegetables, whole grains, high-fiber foods, and unprocessed foods. Increasing your intake of these types of carbohydrates will help control blood sugar, insulin levels, energy levels, and body fat.

Some examples of complex carbs are legumes, beans, whole grains, brown rice pasta, oats, quinoa, and brown rice. We are going to make small changes to your diet that will make a big difference. For example, you can always use brown rice pasta, chickpea pasta, or spaghetti squash instead of regular white pasta because they will help to balance the insulin levels in your body.

The most important point to remember here is that not all carbohydrates are good for your health. For example, you should limit your intake of simple carbs such as fruit juice, candy, table sugar, honey, maple syrup, and soda because they cause a spike in your sugar levels.

When you eat simple carbs, your body converts them into sugar, which enters your bloodstream, where these sugars (glucose) can either be used for immediate energy or stored for later use.

The second-largest component of macronutrients is fats. Although many people try to avoid these, they are very important to maintain a healthy diet! There is a common misconception that fats make you fat, but that is not the case.

Some people are scared to eat fats because they think they will make them gain weight. But the reality is that what makes you gain weight is the excess calorie intake and the kind of fats you consume.

Fats are important because they help balance hormone levels in our brain and nervous system so that they can function properly. Healthy fats help your body to absorb vitamins A, D, E, and K.

If you consume too much fat, your body will convert it into body fat, leading to weight gain and obesity. All fats are high in energy and provide 9 kcal of energy, which is a lot more than the 4 kcal of energy carbs and proteins have.

There are two types of fats—saturated and unsaturated. Most saturated fats come from animal products. However, some of them do not. Coconut oil is a great example. Some other not-so-healthy sources of saturated fats are butter, fatty meats, cheese, and full-fat dairy products.

Unsaturated fats are a healthier choice as they can help to reduce your risk of heart disease and high cholesterol. They are mostly found in plant-based foods and fish, including nuts, seeds, olive oil, salmon, and avocado.

The last and very important component of macronutrients is protein. Protein plays a huge role in balancing the insulin, cholesterol, and hormones of your body, resulting in healthy weight loss. Proteins are made up of amino acids that join to form long chains. They are needed in your diet for the growth and maintenance of different organs, muscles, tissues, bones, skin, and hair. Proteins help to energize your body and carry oxygen throughout the body.

Proteins make antibodies, which fight infections and boost your immunity. Eating proteins also keeps your cells healthy and helps to create new ones. Some major sources of protein include fish, plants, dairy, poultry, lean beef, eggs, seeds, nuts, beans, legumes, and quinoa.

If you want to maintain a healthy weight, then your ideal macronutrient consumption should be approximately 40–50% carbohydrates, 25–30% protein, and 20–25% fat every day.

Another important component of healthy eating is fiber. You need to ensure you are eating the right amount of fiber every day, as it will help to regulate your bowel movements, cleanse your body, and lower your cholesterol levels. Foods that are high in fiber will also help your body fight against constipation, weight gain, diabetes, heart disease, and cancers. A lot of the macros we have just discussed contain a good amount of fiber.

We consume two types of fiber daily—soluble and insoluble. Soluble fiber dissolves in water and forms a gel-like material. It can help lower blood glucose levels and cholesterol, which results in weight loss. On the other hand, insoluble fiber helps to move everything through your digestive system, prevents constipation, and regulates your bowel movements.

Both soluble and insoluble fiber-rich foods keep you full longer and speed up your weight loss. Foods that are high in fiber include oats, apples, beans, lentils, beets, cabbage, and cauliflower.

"We sometimes underestimate the influence of little things."

—Charles W. Chesnutt

What Are Micronutrients?

*M*icronutrients mainly consist of vitamins and minerals. We do not need large amounts of these, which is why they are called "micros." However, they are an integral part of our healthy nutrient intake.

The micronutrients in our bodies help to regulate our metabolism, heartbeat, cellular pH, and bone density. Micronutrient deficiency may lead to diseases like metabolic syndrome, osteoporosis (lack of vitamin D), and obesity.

Micronutrients, such as vitamins, are necessary for energy production, immune function, blood clotting, and other functions in our bodies. In contrast, minerals are responsible for our growth, bone health, fluid balance, and several other processes.

The vitamin micronutrients are found in two forms—water-soluble and fat-soluble. Water-soluble vitamins easily dissolve in water and are harder for your body to store (including vitamin C and the B vitamins).

Some sources of water-soluble vitamins are broccoli, citrus fruits, mango, strawberries, cauliflower, red bell peppers, lettuce, mushrooms, lentils, spinach, yogurt, eggs, and fish. Because they are more difficult for your body to store, they must be included regularly in a healthy diet.

The fat-soluble vitamins get stored in your liver and fatty tissue. These are mainly the vitamins that dissolve well in lipids, for example, vitamins A, D, E, and K. Some of the main sources of fat-soluble vitamins are found in pumpkins, squash, carrots, eggs, melons, sweet potatoes, nuts, and tofu.

"The first wealth
is health."

—Ralph Waldo Emerson

What Should I Keep in My Kitchen to Prepare Healthy Meals?

I always remind my clients that healthy eating comes from what is in your kitchen. Exercise can only take you so far if you keep munching on sugary cheesecakes or pizzas all the time. You also need to eat the right foods.

The list below, which is classified into food groups, includes the main ingredients you should keep in your kitchen if you want to maintain your overall physical and mental health. These include but aren't limited to:

Proteins

- Lean meats
- Fish
- Eggs
- Low-fat yogurt
- Protein powders
- Tofu

Veggies/Fruits

- Spinach
- Broccoli
- Cauliflower
- Mixed berries
- Oranges
- Kale
- Lemons
- Garlic
- Ginger
- Beets
- Carrots
- Celery
- Cucumbers
- Blueberries
- Bananas
- Apples
- Pears
- Strawberries
- Pineapple
- Eggplant
- Zucchini
- Onions
- Pumpkin

Fats

- Nuts
- Avocados
- Extra virgin olive oil
- Flax seeds
- Chia seeds
- Coconut oil
- Almond butter

Carbs

- Oats
- Quinoa
- Beans
- Lentils
- Brown rice
- Sweet potatoes
- Brown rice pasta
- Chickpea pasta

Others

- Salsa
- Tomato sauce
- Honey
- Stevia
- Herbs for seasoning (oregano, dandelion, thyme, rosemary, etc.)
- Hummus
- Seltzer

Eating healthy does not mean you need to sacrifice taste or let go of your favorite foods, but it does mean that you need to find healthy alternatives for your unhealthy foods. You can always season your foods to your taste and enjoy your meals as such!

There are so many ways to customize your diet so you enjoy yourself while making healthier choices. The key is to find out what works best for you.

The following tips might help you in your search for healthier food alternatives:

- Instead of store-bought salad dressings, make your own, use balsamic vinegar, or lemon juice to dress your salads or veggies.

- BBQ, indoor grill, steam, air fry, pressure cook, or bake your food—do not fry!

- Use chicken or vegetable broth to replace oils when cooking.

- Use cooking sprays instead of oil or butter.

- Use skim milk or unsweetened almond, coconut, or cashew milk instead of regular whole milk.

- Prepare your foods and snacks in advance, so you do not munch on unhealthy options when you get hungry.

- Snack on veggies with hummus or salsa.

- Make your own marinades.

- Replace simple carbs with complex carbs (i.e., sweet potato instead of white potato).

- Use stevia instead of sugar in coffee, teas, iced teas, smoothies, oatmeal, etc.

You might think that eating healthier means you need to buy all organic or your grocery bills need to be much higher, but that is not the case. You can eat healthily and keep those bills down.

"Exercise is king.
Nutrition is queen.
Put them together, and
you've got a kingdom."

—Jack LaLanne

Healthy Meals Throughout the Day

*Y*ou need to make sure that you are fueling your body with the right nutrients throughout the day. Your breakfast, lunch, dinner, and snacks need to be balanced to meet your health goals.

A protein-rich breakfast that includes eggs, salmon, low-fat dairy, tofu, or even oatmeal will help to kick-start your metabolism and burn more calories. Protein will also help keep you fuller for longer, so you eat fewer calories the rest of the day.

If you do not feel like eating in the morning, go for a protein shake. You can simply add your favorite protein powder to the blender with some fruits to make a delicious protein shake or smoothie. Similarly, you can top your morning toast with a scrambled egg, an omelet, avocado, or hummus.

For your lunch or dinner, you can always go for veggies, chicken, fish, fiber-rich foods, or complex carbs. This will keep your energy and insulin levels in check and get you through the day. You need to choose the carbs that produce a steady rise in blood sugar, which means cutting out white foods (white rice, white bread, regular pasta) and munching on high-fiber foods instead.

Good high-fiber foods are beans, legumes, brown pasta, green veggies, and quinoa. Do not cut off carbs completely because they are low in fat and rich in fiber. The key is to combine carbs with healthy essential fats, like salmon and mackerel, or nuts and seeds like flax, chia, or pumpkin. Your body will use these healthy fats alongside the protein to regenerate and repair the important cells required for healthy skin, hair, and nails.

As mentioned in the previous section, I would also recommend that you maintain a food diary or journal to write down everything you eat. This way, you know that you're absorbing the essential nutrients you need every day from all the healthy and clean foods that you eat.

Make changes at your own pace, so you do not feel overwhelmed. Take one step at a time and understand that this journey requires a lot of consistency and motivation. Try to be as happy and stress-free as possible to keep yourself motivated. Surround yourself with positive-minded people who are ready to support you in your weight loss and overall health journey.

Do not forget to smile and eat right, even on your busiest days. It is going to give you immense energy and motivation to stay on track. All you need to do is have faith in yourself and believe that you have the power to create change. The rest will fall into place in no time!

PART THREE
Stress & Sleep

"The only journey is the journey within."

—Rainer Maria Rilke

What Is Good
Mental Health?

*M*ichelle had a goal in mind. She wanted to fit into the dress she'd bought for her brother's wedding and wanted a certain weight to appear on that scale. So, she decided to follow a crash diet that promised her the results she was eagerly seeking.

Michelle ate very little. She ignored the hunger pangs and the reduced energy levels she was experiencing. Overall, she felt very irritable. She had done this several times before. You may be able to relate.

As the wedding drew closer and Michelle was not hitting all of her goals, she started to feel like a failure. She had a lot of negative thoughts about herself, and she believed something was wrong with her. But the truth is, she is not a failure. *And you are not a failure either!*

Often, we just don't realize that our bodies are talking to us. We have learned to ignore many of the signs it sends us, and we have learned to judge ourselves in a lot of negative ways.

We fixate on that number staring back at us from the scale. I don't want you to focus on a number, but rather, focus on how you feel inside as well as on the outside.

If you start to listen to your body, connect with it, ask it what it needs in the moment, what it needs for the future to stay healthy, and stop with that number on the scale, then you will be able to free yourself from the negative self-talk. Remind yourself how amazing you are, how important you are to yourself and others around you.

Balancing our mental health is such an important aspect of our overall health. Good mental health can be recognized as taking care of your body and knowing how/when to listen to your body. (The mind and body are so connected!) Making healthy choices/habits daily will help maintain your overall healthy lifestyle.

One thing I always say to my clients and family is this: LISTEN TO YOUR BODY! Your body knows best when it is being pushed too hard or not hard enough. It sends you signs when you need to slow down or push harder.

So, even if you have not been listening to the signs that your body has been sending, the good news is that it's not too late! You can start listening now and get yourself in a happier, healthier place.

I do understand that sometimes it is easier said than done, and many times it is hard to put your needs first. But when it comes to your health, you need to remind yourself that it is ok to take care of your health and work on your own self-acceptance!

These signs come in all different ways. For example, if you are really tired, you may feel irritable, less focused, or your eye may twitch. Sometimes when you are pushing yourself too hard at the gym, you may feel nauseous, and then you know it is time to hold back a little.

Along your journey, your body and mind will be saying things to you all the time. Some will be awesome, like the extra energy you are feeling from making positive changes, and other times it may be a feeling of disappointment, like the low you're experiencing because you chose to eat cake instead of fruit at a party.

It is very important that you stay positive and keep telling yourself that you are worth it! Everyone makes mistakes, we are human and sometimes we go off on different paths until we get back on the right one.

Remind yourself that you are strong and you can do this. Go back to why you started this journey to become healthier. When you start to lose your focus, just remind yourself that you are working toward the best version of yourself!

Some important choices/habits to consider:

- Getting adequate sleep
- Eating a balanced healthy diet
- Practicing a fitness/exercise routine
- Spending time with good, positive friends
- Incorporating meditation (even if for five minutes a day)
- Journaling
- Setting SMART goals

- Making a Pinterest board
- Getting fresh air
- Creating daily routines
- Forgiving yourself—no one is perfect, failure is a stepping stone to success when you learn from it
- Investing in yourself
- Laughing! Remember, laughter is the best medicine!
- Respecting yourself!
- Celebrating *you* because you ROCK!

I find making a Pinterest board of my favorite quotes, songs, recipes, and workout clothing all help to keep me motivated. I keep it somewhere that I can see daily. Sometimes I put them in my kitchen, on my phone, or somewhere that I know I will see them as daily reminders.

I also like to share them with friends (especially the recipes) so we can cook together or share the healthy dishes we have made. This also helps me stay connected to my friends who are on their own health journey.

Many of my clients have also tried this and find it helpful. They laugh with their friends, learn healthy recipes, and even meet their friends to walk and share fun stories.

"Every day brings a choice:
To practice stress,
or to practice peace."

—Joan Borysenko

Stress Management

Stress has become a major problem for many people—a hectic job, chaotic home life, uncontrolled finances, and bad habits such as unhealthy eating, drinking, and smoking all contribute to adversely high stress levels.

According to Cleveland Clinic, stress is a normal reaction that everyone experiences, and our bodies are designed to respond to it. Stress is not always a bad thing, but it can be bad if your body does not get relief or relaxation.

Unfortunately, we all experience stress in some way, but everyone perceives stress differently. Something that you may find stressful may not seem stressful to someone else. We cannot fully eliminate all of the stress from our lives, but we can learn how to cope with it and handle it in ways that can help calm us down.

I want to share a story about one of my clients and how handling her stress has helped her.

Sarah has two beautiful kids and a full-time job. She is married, but her husband works long hours and is not around during the week to help with the daily needs of their kids. Handling two kids while working full-time can be extremely stressful at times.

Sarah came to me and asked for guidance on how she could possibly fit exercise or "me time" into her already hectic life. She explained that she is driving carpools, helping with homework, making meals, and running errands, all while working full-time. But she felt so stressed out that she needed help with strategies to handle her stress.

We worked together on finding a few ways to help with the stress and help her breathe a little easier. The first thing I asked her to do was download a breathing/meditation app on her phone. She was very skeptical about this and said she was not someone who "did this."

I asked her to *just try* while she was sitting in the car for five minutes, just five minutes while she was waiting for the kids to come out of practice. I suggested that she listen to the guided app on breathing/meditation one or two times and let me know how it went.

The first time, she was just doing it to just make me happy, but then she realized it actually helped to calm her down and feel more focused. I was so glad to hear this!

Sarah now takes three to five minutes daily in the car to stop and breathe. As we worked together, we also came up with a plan for fitting in some exercise and healthy eating tips, which also helped her stress levels feel more manageable.

And now, Sarah is sleeping better and feels more rested!

On a side note, the guided app has also helped many other people I know, including some of my kids' teenage/college-age friends. Seriously, give it a try!

Excessive stress and tension contribute to numerous physical and mental health problems such as high blood pressure, cardiovascular disease, muscle tension, headaches, diabetes, chronic depression, obesity, and fatigue. The list continues with other chronic health problems and mental health diagnoses.

However, before we go into further details about the causes and effects of stress, we need to know what stress is. Stress is a feeling of emotional or physical tension that can come from any event or thought. These events or thoughts often make you feel frustrated, angry, or nervous. **Stress is your body's reaction to a challenge or demand.**

What Are the Most Common Effects of Stress?

Stress can be the root cause of many of our physical and mental health problems. Some of the most common effects of stress include:

Fatigue: Stress can make you feel tired, sleepy, and dizzy—even after getting an adequate amount of sleep. Excessive stress can make these symptoms worse. With fatigue, your muscles are sore and weak and there is pain throughout your body. Sometimes, fatigue will make you unreasonably moody and irritated. Irritability and anxiety lead to multiple sleep and eating disorders, such as overeating, under-eating, or excessive sleeping.

Headache: One of the most common triggers of tension-type headaches and migraines is stress. It is a tension headache if there are light sensations of tightness or pressure on the sides or back of your head or across your forehead. Some people experience tenderness on their scalp, neck, or shoulder muscles alongside a dull, aching head pain.

Diabetes: It is possible that there may be a link between stress and your risk of developing Type 2 diabetes. High levels of stress hormones in your body may stop insulin-producing cells in your pancreas from working properly, thus reducing the amount of insulin they make. By focusing on lowering your stress levels and the tension in your body caused by stress, you can reverse some of these effects on your blood sugar and insulin sensitivity.

Heart Disease: High levels of cortisol (one of the body's stress hormones) can increase blood cholesterol, triglycerides, blood sugar, and blood pressure. Long-term stress increases the levels of cortisol in your body and can also cause a buildup of plaque deposits in your arteries. High levels of cortisol and a buildup of plaque in your arteries are two of the main risk factors associated with heart disease.

Obesity: There is a very strong connection between obesity and stress for several reasons.

- First, chronic stress leads to comfort eating, which often involves the overeating of high-fat, high-sugar, and high-calorie foods, which in turn leads to weight gain.

- Second, people with chronic stress do not feel motivated to work out or exercise on a regular basis, which again contributes to weight gain.

- Third, people with more stress can suffer from hormonal imbalances, different types of nutrient deficiencies, water retention, and bloating.

These will all lead to excessive weight gain. Whether the stress makes you overeat unhealthy foods, cease to work out regularly, or provides the fuel for the hormonal imbalances and bloating, this weight gain can eventually lead to obesity.

"Fitness isn't about
looking good, it is about
feeling unstoppable,
strong, badass, and beautiful
in your own skin."

—Unknown

Maintaining Good
Mental Health

Your mental health affects how you think, feel, and act as you go through life. It also affects how you handle stress, relate to others, and make decisions. To live a stress-reduced life, you need to make sure that your mind is happy and healthy as consistently as possible.

In the thirty years of my health and fitness career, I have seen how clients and friends who suffer from anxiety and depression have a comparatively harder time coping with stress than others who do not suffer from anxiety and depression. It is difficult for those who struggle with these mental health disorders to think about anything positive when they are facing so much negativity each and every day. Before they can face the stress in their life, I advise them to work on their mental health. Sometimes, they need to find a therapist who can help further.

Here, I will highlight some of the most common techniques to maintain good mental health.

Exercise Regularly: Exercise reduces levels of cortisol and adrenaline (the body's stress hormones). Exercise also stimulates the production of endorphins—natural chemicals in the brain (endogenous) that are the body's painkillers. Endorphins are also mood elevators and when your body releases them, your stress levels go down. When you exercise, you are going to feel better, more confident, and like you have accomplished something. You will feel like you can get through tougher days because your brain is clearer and therefore able to process things in your everyday life.

Practice Mindfulness: Sometimes, we feel down or depressed because we think about something from our past or what our future will look like. Mindfulness can serve the purpose of helping you slow down enough to focus on what you are feeling and on what you are sensing in the present moment, moving you out of judgment and stress and into peace and calm. It is a form of meditation that uses breathing techniques and guided imagery to relax the body and center you in peace with what *is*.

Get Seven Hours of Sleep: It has been proven that the most effective stress reducer is getting enough sleep. When you get enough sleep, your body's stress levels decline, and you can better cope with stress. Following a regular sleep routine will calm and restore your body, improve your concentration, and regulate your mood.

Stay Positive (Think Healthy, Be Healthy): We all know that it is nearly impossible to have a stress-free life. The good news is there are ways to cope with your stress. I believe that staying positive in stressful situations is important when it comes to coping with stress. Positive thinking can do wonders for your mental and physical health. It can help reduce your stress level, make you feel better about yourself (or the situation), and improve your overall well-being and outlook.

Participate in Activities That You Enjoy: Who doesn't love fun movie nights or hanging out with friends? People who are involved in more fun activities are less likely to be depressed. Having regular fun in your life can help you feel less overwhelmed by the stressors you face. Daily or weekly fun activities can help your body to release endorphins and increase the levels of serotonin in your body. Serotonin is a hormone associated with making you feel better.

I find it to be helpful to actually schedule in fun as though it is an item on your weekly (or even daily) to-do list. Make yourself relax into enjoyment because when you set aside the time, you'll actually feel productive while having a good time, rather than feeling guilt or shame for taking time away from what you "should" be doing. This will help you change the attitude you have toward your life's stressors so that you are less reactive to stress when you do experience it.

Get Some Sunshine: Have you ever noticed how your mood gets better on a gloomy day when the sun starts to peek through the clouds? Well, there's a reason behind that. Sunlight increases the brain's release of serotonin, which helps a person feel calmer and happier. Spending some time in the sun every day can help reduce your stress levels while helping you to feel fresh, awake, and ready to tackle the challenges of the day.

Unplug from Your Devices: Although it is essential for us to have a healthy relationship with technology because it is such an important part of our world, anything in excess can harm our health—it is the same with technology. Do you check your work email at the dinner table or when you are out with friends or family? Do you constantly scroll through social media? These could be signs that you need to unplug from your devices for a period of time each day.

Unfortunately, the constant use of electronic devices like cell phones, laptops, tablets, televisions, and computers can disrupt your mental and physical health. Overusing technology causes stress, loneliness, anxiety, physical ailments, and sleep deprivation. Your brain and body need to recover from your day at work.

Being *on* 24/7 is neither healthy for your mind, your body, nor your spirit. If during every break you take, you are on a screen, then you are on it for too much time each day. You need to take time out of your day for yourself—sans technology. Instead, take this time to reconnect with your loved ones.

Unplug from work-related technology after work hours. Once you get home, technology for work use should stop. In fact, all technology use should stop, at least for a moment. Block out a screen-free time period each day for your household. It will make you feel much more relaxed and calm.

"More smiling, less worrying.
More compassion, less judgment.
More blessed, less stressed.
More love, less hate."

—Roy T. Bennett

Coping with Stress

*R*ecently, one of my friends posted on her Instagram, "If stress could burn calories, I'd be a supermodel." I found that funny. Your stress attacks your body as soon as you open your eyes in the morning and stays with you until you go to sleep at night.

Nowadays, most people have become so stressed because of their hectic schedules and busy lifestyles that they hardly get time for themselves. They keep getting stressed over little things, and it is their routine that is to blame for this stress.

We often get stressed over little things, like not getting a phone call from a close friend on our birthday, getting sudden acne, or seeing something on social media that we were not invited to, etc. All these things bother us because we are already stressed out about something else from earlier in the day or from the day before.

Once you become stressed or tense about something, everything else starts irritating you too. It is a chain reaction that your body feels. For example, if you wake up late or miss your bus in the morning, you already have a stressor at the start of your day. After a morning like that, even the little things will irritate you throughout your day.

What if, instead of allowing waking up late or missing the bus to be a stressor, you brush it off and do not let it bother you? If you do that, any other small thing will not irritate you as much because you are now in a more positive mental state.

Apart from exercising and getting enough sleep, practicing relaxation techniques like deep breathing, guided meditation, and getting massages can also help you to lower your stress levels. I tell my clients that they need to take some time out of the day for themselves so they have the time to practice exercises, yoga, relaxation, and stretching techniques. These physical workouts and practices have proven benefits for your mental health and stress management.

Another important thing to remember about stress management is that you don't need to isolate yourself. You should go out and interact with other people, even if you are feeling down or depressed. Your social circle can have a big impact on your mood. Make sure that you are surrounded by happy, positive, uplifting people as much as possible.

You want to stay away from people with negative vibes who cause you stress. There is a saying about crabby people—misery loves company. *If they can't have it, neither can you.* People get jealous when they see others achieving their goals. They are not as successful, so they try to keep you down or sabotage you from reaching your goals.

Try to spend more time with your family and friends who build you up and cheer you up when you are down. Whenever you are feeling down or stressed, do not hesitate to ask for help.

There is nothing wrong with getting social support, as it can help you to feel relaxed and much more at peace.

Just like our bodies, our minds also need food to survive. **I believe that the best food for our mind is happiness**. You need to engage in all the activities that make you feel happy. For example, you can go out and party with your friends, enjoy a movie night, go for a walk with your loved one, or bake some cookies for yourself. Taking this time every day will boost your mood and energy levels.

WebMD estimates that 75%-90% of all doctor visits are related to stress. Isn't that percentage a bit too high? It certainly is. My point is that you don't need to carry all of this stress in your life because there are solutions to help reduce it or cope with it.

If you are truly trying to have a happier, healthier life, then you need to make sure that your routine is as healthy and as stress-free as possible. An organized schedule can help you with mental calmness, psychological comfort, and relaxation.

If you feel, at this stage of your life, that you are stressed and yet you are not engaging in any regular physical activity, get up and start now because *it is never too late*. You will fall in love with your transformation *inside and out* once you get started. And to make the process easier, here are some tips that will help you to design a stress-free daily schedule.

- Make a list of what you need to do for the day/week at the beginning of your day/week.

- Structure the list using morning/early, morning/late, afternoon/late, afternoon/evening.

- Prioritize your list and put it in order of priority (commit to the time when the particular to-do list item will get done).

- Take time out for your friends and family, fun, self-care, exercise, and meal prep.

- Put at least seven hours of sleep each night on your schedule.

- Make a vision board. It will be immensely helpful in allowing you to see your end goals and the reasons why you are doing each of these things every day.

I also recommend you have a journal for writing daily thoughts, logging exercise, and tracking your food. The journal will help you analyze the causes of your stress.

"Don't be pushed around
by the fears in your mind.
Be led by the dreams
in your heart.."

—Roy T. Bennett

Positive Affirmations

In your daily journal, include positive affirmations. Personally, I love positive affirmations and I strongly believe in them. My positive affirmation is: *SHE BELIEVED SHE COULD, SO SHE DID!* Every day, I say this to myself and keep repeating it so that I am motivated all day long, to move toward achieving my goals.

There are numerous examples of positive affirmations that you can include in your daily journal and in your life, such as:

- I can and I will.
- I have the power to create change.
- I believe in the person I am becoming.
- I am my own superhero.
- I approve of myself and love myself deeply and completely.
- I choose to be proud of myself.
- With every breath I take, I release stress from my body.
- Happiness is my choice.
- I am the powerhouse; I am indestructible!

- The greatest responsibility is to love yourself and to know you are enough.

I believe that we should live every moment to the fullest and become the best version of ourselves. Living a healthy and happy life is your birthright. Stay positive and know that you are worth it! Remember that taking time out for yourself when it comes to health is not being selfish! You need to do this to stay mentally and physically healthy!

"Good company on a journey
makes the way seem shorter."

—Izaak Walton

How to Form a Proper Sleep Schedule

*D*octors recommend getting at least seven hours of undisturbed and peaceful sleep every day. Good sleep helps you improve your concentration levels and focus and helps regulate your hormones, weight, and immune system. It also takes care of your emotional well-being and reduces your stress levels. If you get the right amount of sleep, you are in a better state of mind to deal with any daily stressors you face.

Sometimes we cannot control the factors that limit the amount of sleep we get. We might have things going on at work that stress us out. We might have family stress, health issues, or other things on our minds.

But there are some ways we can improve our sleep so we can get a proper and peaceful night's sleep:

- Stick to a daily schedule. Go to bed and wake up at the same time every day (even on weekends).
- If you do not fall asleep within twenty minutes, get out of bed and do something relaxing like listening to calming music or deep breathing.
- Avoid caffeine late in the day.
- Limit naps.

- Exercise daily.
- Eat healthily.
- Do not drink too much liquid close to bedtime.
- Create a calm, peaceful environment where you sleep.

Apart from eating healthy, exercising, staying positive, and getting proper sleep, make sure that you surround yourself with positive and optimistic people. It will help you accomplish your health goals.

Stay away from toxic behaviors and negative people. Both will create hurdles for you or demotivate you on your health journey, and you may find it difficult to get adequate sleep as a result.

At the end of the day, you need to remember that a healthy mental state is the biggest asset you can have. No matter how healthily you eat or exercise, if you do not feel happy on the inside and those around you do not support you, then it will be very hard for you to succeed.

Say to yourself, "I believe in the person I am becoming! I can do anything I put my mind to, and I am stronger than I think!" Consider writing this on a sticky note and putting it on your bathroom mirror to remind yourself of it.

Living a healthy lifestyle is not hard, it just takes time to adjust. When you do, there will be no reason to look back. You will feel better about yourself, inside and out!

PART FOUR
Fitness

Toughness is in the soul and
spirit, not in the muscles.
YOU GOT THIS !

What Is Considered a Healthy Fitness Routine?

*N*utritionists and trainers get asked all the time, "How can I include exercise in my daily routine?" The answer is simple. You need motivation and mental focus. That's it!

Exercising is extremely important for everyone to incorporate into their daily lives, whether you are a child, a teenager, or an older woman. Understanding the significance of incorporating physical activity into our lives will help us pay equal attention to it as we would any other daily tasks, such as brushing our teeth or taking a shower.

Thirty to forty minutes of exercise in your daily routine is vital for your overall well-being. A healthy fitness routine consists of aerobic fitness, strength training, core exercises, balance, flexibility, and stretching. To practice any of these aspects of a healthy fitness routine, you have two options—either you can hit the gym or do regular workouts at home.

A full-fledged workout is not necessarily what you always have to be going for. Small activities like walking, jogging, yoga, or dance can all serve the same purpose—keeping a healthy fitness routine. You don't have to stress yourself out if one of the exercises seems too much for you. If you think the exercise is not suitable for you, instead of forcing yourself to do it, choose to practice one of the other types of physical activity.

Some of my clients want to start running, but since they have not been running, they need to start slowly with a combination of walking and running. Day by day, they increase their running time and decrease the walking time in their workouts. Other clients may not have as much time and want to incorporate strength and cardio in their thirty minutes, so I suggest HIIT training for them.

The American College of Sports Medicine recommends thirty minutes of physical activity five times a week to stay healthy and fit. They explain that regular and consistent exercise helps you by:

- Controlling your weight
- Reducing your risk of cardiovascular diseases
- Stabilizing your blood sugar/insulin levels
- Improving your mental health/mood
- Improving your concentration levels, judgment skills, and focus
- Strengthening your bones
- Reducing your chance of osteoporosis
- Reducing your risk of certain cancers
- Giving you better balance (reducing the risk of falls)
- Improving your sleep

Many people who know me know that I workout to not only stay fit and reap all of the above-listed benefits but for my mental health, as well! It is my stress reliever, my therapy. It puts me in a good mood, and it keeps the structure of my day.

When I am having a bad day or really just need to escape from my crazy life, I work out. It helps to clear my mind. I do my best thinking and come up with so many ideas and solutions during my workouts.

I can also say that when it is time to go to sleep, I rarely have a hard time falling asleep, and exercise definitely plays a role in that. Exercising regularly has also helped to build my self-confidence and self-esteem. I feel as strong on the inside as I do on the outside.

One of the most important reasons to consider a healthy fitness routine is for YOU! Make sure you are doing this for yourself and not for someone else. This is the only way it will truly work. Keep your mind open and remember that you can do anything you put your mind to!

"Motivation is what gets you started. Habit is what keeps you going."

—Jim Rohn

How to Start or Get Back into Your Exercise Routine

*T*here are days when you are in vacation mode or don't feel like working out. Maybe you have too much work on your plate. Maybe you are stressed or depressed. Maybe you claim you don't have enough time or motivation to engage in physical activity.

It is normal to have some of those days, everybody has them. However, you cannot surrender to that line of thinking. Instead, when those thought patterns arise, you need to push yourself to take some time out of your day to exercise, even if it is walking around your neighborhood.

Starting a new exercise routine or getting back to your previous one is not as difficult as it may seem. There are two steps, but first, you need to promise yourself that you will stay consistent with your workouts. If this is not your first time getting back into exercise, you need to tell yourself that you won't give up this time. Say to yourself, "I have the power to create change."

First, you need to set **SMART** goals for yourself. That is, your exercise goals should be Specific, Measurable, Attainable, Relevant, and Timely (SMART). For instance, this week, I will walk twenty minutes for five days. This goal is (S) specific, can be (M) measured in terms of time and days, is (A) achievable, is (R) relevant because it is working toward my goal of developing a healthier lifestyle, is bound to a one-week period and therefore, (T) timely.

Do not set unachievable goals for yourself. When starting out, set short, attainable goals for one week or one day at a time. Your goal must be defined in a way that is specific and allows you to measure it to see if you were successful in completing your goal.

If you set goals that are unachievable, you will only end up disappointed. It is also important to make sure that your goals are relevant to your life and what you ultimately want to accomplish.

Go easy on yourself and decide what types of workouts you can realistically incorporate into your health routine. You are the best judge and decision-maker for yourself because nobody understands *you* better than you do. Keep all the external negative people and attitudes away, decide what suits you, and go with it.

Second, put your specific workouts on your daily schedule and make it fun! Make sure that you are taking time out every day for exercising and that you are consistent with it. Keep motivating yourself through every workout because there is no guarantee that you will have other people to motivate you.

Share your workouts on social media! Post your workout pictures and videos everywhere, like Facebook, Instagram, TikTok, or Twitter. You will show people that you are having fun, you will get more support, and you will feel like participating in more physical activity.

Remember, those who make you feel good about yourself are the *keepers*, and it will benefit you to spend more time with them. In the end, you need to be your own best friend and cheerleader.

You will need to start slowly and listen to your body. Initially, you should do light to moderate workouts. Then, you should gradually increase your workout's intensity.

In the first week, you should start with lighter weights, modifying your cardio by not doing all high-impact training, and even when sore, commit to doing a workout every day. If you skip a day or two because you are sore, you will continue this pattern.

Then, before you know it, you will only be working out twice a week and you will have lost all your progress. But, if you work out even when sore in the first week, you will get through the worst part and will not be as sore moving forward.

After a few weeks, you will notice that you are feeling stronger and will be able to push yourself more. Maybe that means adding in heavier weights, doing more reps, or being able to modify less on cardio.

My experience shows that within a week, you will feel a boost. Within about two weeks, you'll start to notice a significant improvement in your energy levels, concentration, and blood circulation. You'll experience fewer mood swings and less irritability. Once your body gets into the habit of exercising, it will start to consistently feel great, and you will feel like working out more. It is a positive feedback cycle.

The last but most important thing to remember is that you are exercising for yourself. You are not working out for anybody else. You will see it all come together when you exercise with *your* end goal in mind, not someone else's.

Believe in yourself and remind yourself why you are doing this. Ask yourself, *What benefits am I going to get by exercising?* You know the benefits are all positive. Exercising for yourself will bring out so much motivation that you will no doubt continue to work out and keep up your healthy lifestyle.

"Exercise should be regarded as a tribute to the heart."

—Gene Tunney

How Can I Be Physically Active Throughout the Day?

*U*sing these tips, you will be able to engage in more regular physical activity.

1. Make your daily routine activities *more* active. Make sure you stand up and walk around your house from time to time, listen to your favorite song and turn it into a dance party, or take your dog for a longer-than-usual walk.

2. Be active with others—go for a walk, a hike, or join a fitness center with a friend.

3. Make it FUN and post your progress on social media or take a before picture to stay motivated and track your progress.

4. Track your progress in a daily log to feel more accomplished or to hold yourself accountable for daily workouts.

5. Be consistent with your workouts. Don't skip your exercise on stressful days or on days where you feel like you cannot find time for yourself. These days are so

important to get something in because it will make you feel more energized in the end.

6. Do not sit for more than an hour. Take a walk around the house or around your office space at work to feel more active. Set an alarm to make sure you are up and moving every hour.

"To enjoy the glow of
good health, you must exercise."

—Gene Tunney

Exercise

*E*xercise is not just about weight loss, bodybuilding, or toning. It's also about improving the quality of your overall mental, emotional, and physical wellbeing. Women who engage in regular workouts reap amazing benefits, like a toned body, better sleep, glowing skin, faster metabolism, and improved mental health.

According to the American Academy of Family Physicians, regular exercise can lower your blood pressure, help to maintain healthy weight and cholesterol levels, and prevent chronic health issues like diabetes and cardiovascular disease. A daily thirty-minute workout session can be enough for you to improve your cognitive function, immunity, and overall physical and mental health.

Jordan Horowitz, M.D., a gynecologist with Sutter Pacific Medical Foundation and clinical professor at the University of California, says, "When we think of healthcare, we often focus on doctor visits, preventive care, lab tests, and immunizations. But other factors are in our personal control, like improving our diets, reducing stress, and adding fun to our lives. Exercise is one of these controllable factors, and it's highly effective at improving health."

This is so true! I believe that most of our health issues can be improved easily with the help of regular exercise and physical activity.

If you have health issues like diabetes, high blood pressure, PCOS, or obesity, then you should form a steady workout routine and stick to it rather than being on medication for your entire life. Exercise is not a luxury but a necessity.

Exercise is as important as your other chores like brushing your teeth, combing your hair, or making your bed right after getting up in the morning. Gone are the days when workouts were considered something fancy or extra. Nowadays, exercise has become necessary for all of us because of our modern and inactive lifestyles.

Exercising is for everyone! However, before starting any exercise program, never forget to consult your doctor.

As we have already discussed the health benefits of regular exercise, it is time for us now to discuss the different types of exercise. Exercise is usually grouped into four categories: endurance (cardio), strength, flexibility, and balance.

One of the best ways to get into the exercising spirit is to listen to your favorite music. Music can be therapeutic and fun as it boosts your mood and brings back good memories. It can be motivating when doing endurance or cardio, or it can be extra calming and soothing—especially if you are working on flexibility, yoga, or Pilates.

"Don't let anyone work
harder than you do."

—Serena Williams

What Is Cardio?

*T*he term cardio is short for cardiovascular exercises. It is a movement that gets your heart rate up and increases the blood circulation throughout your body for a certain period. Doing cardio will help you burn fat when you combine it with proper nutrition. While doing a cardio workout, our goal is to get our heart rate up to our target heart rate (THR) or higher rate of perceived exertion (RPE).

Cardio workouts can help women to develop bone mass density, lose weight, speed up their metabolism, prevent chronic diseases, boost mental health, and improve hormonal balance. Regular cardio workouts also play a vital role in uplifting our mood, rejuvenating our skin, and promoting better sleep. However, to reap the full benefits of cardio, you need to stick to a healthy diet plan because you will see quicker results.

To find the perfect type of cardio for yourself, you will need to decide what percent of THR or RPE you want to be at. For example, if I am going for a steady run, my heart rate should be around 60–85% of my maximum heart rate. Normally, you are at 60–70% during warm-ups, 70–80% for the main part of your run, and for harder climbs or sprints, you may be at 80–95%.

You might be wondering what your maximum heart rate is. Well, the formula ACSM uses is 220 minus your age. You then take that number and multiply it by the percentage you are aiming for. For example, if you are forty years old, your maximum heart rate would not be more than 180. You would then multiply 180 by 0.70 to find your target heart rate at 70%, and you would get 126 bpm (beats per minute).

If you are doing a HIIT (High-Intensity Interval Training), then your heart rate will not be steady. If you do not want to calculate your heart rate, you can always use the RPE scale of 1-10. One is the easiest, and ten is the hardest. While doing steady cardio, you will ideally stay between 7 and 8.

"A bear, however
hard he tries,
grows tubby
without exercise."

—A.A. Milne

Common Types of Cardio Exercises:

*H*ere is a list of exercises that will help you elevate your heart rate and increase your blood circulation:

- Running
- Walking
- Swimming
- Zumba/Dance
- Cycling
- Kickboxing
- Elliptical
- Stair climbing
- Jump rope
- Rowing
- Sports
- Kayaking
- Paddleboarding
- Group fitness classes

"If it's easy, then you're doing it wrong."

—Gabby Williams

What Is Strength Training?

Strength training, also known as resistance training, includes particular physical exercises that are designed to improve strength and endurance in men and women. Although mostly associated with weightlifting, strength training comes in a variety of other forms.

Strength training can provide you with significant functional benefits such as improving your overall physical and mental health, increasing bone, muscle, tendon, and ligament strength, improving joint function, and increasing your metabolism and total weight loss.

Strength training also helps in balancing your body and reducing the risk of falls. Regular training like weightlifting and using resistance bands or tubes can help manage chronic conditions such as arthritis, back pain, obesity, heart disease, depression, and diabetes. Although there are many options to choose from when doing strength training, I am highlighting the most common ones here.

> **Body weight:** Use your own body weight to increase the effectiveness of exercises like push-ups, pull-ups, squats, and lunges.

Resistance tubes/bands: An inexpensive and great way to do strength/resistance training. You can find a variety of bands on the market, from low to heavy. Choose according to your body type and goal.

Free weights: Dumbbells can help make you leaner and stronger, and can also tighten the loose skin around your arms, thighs, back, and core.

Weight machines: Most fitness centers offer different machines that you can use to take your workout to the next level—for example, seated arm press, leg curl, or rear leg extension.

Medicine balls: You can use this weighted ball to help level up in conditioning and strength training.

There are so many options at the gym, and most of them turn out to be good so long as you are working under the supervision of a professional gym trainer. Just pick whichever one works best for you.

Sometimes you may even switch things up for fun! I do a lot of my own bodyweight exercises and incorporate free weights, medicine balls, or resistance bands into my workout routine. I like to mix it up to keep my workouts from getting boring and to keep my muscles guessing what is coming next.

Make sure you switch up your workouts. Some days you may want to go for a walk or jog with a friend, or you may want to go by yourself, listening to your favorite tunes. Other days you might want to take a fun Zumba class or get in the water to paddleboard.

A HIIT workout can also incorporate strength training so that you can benefit from both types of exercises in one workout! Isn't that amazing?

The key is always to keep it fun and stay consistent!

"Strength doesn't come from what you can do. It comes from overcoming the things you once thought you couldn't."

—Ashley Greene

HIIT: High-Intensity Interval Training

*H*IIT has become very popular over the past few years, although it's been around much longer than that. HIIT is when you have short bursts of high-intensity exercises combined with short periods of rest or low-intensity exercises. For example, you can sprint for 30 seconds, then walk for 30 seconds.

There are numerous benefits of doing HIIT workouts, but the most known is how you can work out for a shorter period and still burn the same, if not more, calories and fat than a steady, longer cardio workout. And you will also continue to burn calories and lose fat hours after you are done (which you do not get with a steady cardio workout).

The high-intensity part of HIIT is the key component of the workout. You need to push yourself to your maximum intensity (level 9–10, RPE = 9–10, THR = 90% or higher) to get the results. Studies have shown that you can get results in shorter periods of exercise, even just 10–15 minutes.

The Interval part of HIIT is equally important, as it is your rest or active recovery phase. This is when your heart rate starts to come back down. It will go high, then low, which is what makes this type of workout different from steady cardio.

The best part of HIIT workouts is that you will not only burn calories and fat during your workout, but you will continue to burn it off hours after you have finished, due to the afterburn of EPOC (Excess Post-Oxygen Consumption). EPOC is basically the increased levels of oxygen your body consumes and calories it burns to recover from your workout.

"The sweat is the footprint
toward a better you."

—Anonymous

Benefits of Cardio and Strength Training

Many women who've recently broken or fractured a bone think they need to stay away from exercising. That's not true. They should be doing weight-bearing exercises to strengthen their bones so it doesn't happen again. Overall, your exercise routine should include weight-bearing, resistance, and balance exercises.

Prevents Bone Loss and Osteoporosis

Brenda had a bone density test which showed she was at risk for osteoporosis. She did weight-bearing exercises for six straight months, and her follow-up bone density report showed improvement! She was really excited to confirm that exercising was helping her in so many unexpected ways.

Researchers have found that women are more vulnerable to osteoporosis, bone fracture, and height loss than men because they have thinner bones. According to the National Osteoporosis Foundation, "Being female puts you at risk of developing osteoporosis and broken bones."

About half of the women who are above age fifty have a greater risk of breaking a bone. Women lose bone strength more rapidly as they age due to the loss of estrogen in their bodies.

Most aged women with osteoporosis will suffer from a hip fracture and stooped posture due to bone loss. Gratefully, osteoporosis can be prevented through the right type of cardio and strength-training exercises. Your physical activity can help you build strong bones and muscles that stay with you as you age. According to Dr. Horowitz, "During the teen and young adult years is when women build most of the bone mass that can protect them from osteoporosis later in life."

Cardio, resistance, and strength training exercises promote bone health—regardless of age or gender. Jumping rope, weightlifting, kayaking, hiking, aerobics, and jogging build bones and keep them strong. Lifting weights, using exercise bands, squats, planks, or just standing up and rising to your toes will help you to build strength, balance, and flexibility.

Always make sure to talk to your doctor, physical trainer, or gym instructor before starting any new exercises, of course. They can guide you to the safest exercises for your age and condition.

Improves Hormonal Imbalance and Mood Swings

From our first menstrual cycle until menopause, women experience a noticeable change in estrogen and progesterone levels. Various phases of our menstrual cycle affect fertility patterns, brain chemistry, and moods in different ways. Therefore, as women, we need to take extra care of our health routine.

The estrogen levels in a woman's body drop before and during her monthly menstrual cycle as well as leading up to menopause, which decreases the production of serotonin. This dip in serotonin levels makes women more prone to moodiness, depression, and anxiety.

However, the good news is that you can easily deal with mood swings and anxiety if you engage in regular workouts. Cardio exercises can help you to manage these hormonally-triggered mood swings by releasing endorphins into your body, thereby supporting the regulation of your mood.

Some people call it a *runner's high* because endorphins make you feel happy and relaxed after a workout session. "People who experience a runner's high also report feeling less anxiety and reduced pain and they say they feel calmer and happier after exercise," according to *Healthline's* Kimberly Holland.

Reduces Excess Body Fat and Appearance of Cellulite

Women are at a higher risk of gaining weight as they age. As discussed earlier, this could be due to numerous factors, such as a hormonal imbalance, nutrient deficiencies, water retention, pregnancy, or genetics.

Most young women find it extremely difficult to get rid of their excess body fat and cellulite after pregnancy. Some middle-aged women struggle with their weight loss after menopause as they lose estrogen, which in turn, causes their body to redistribute fat cells to their belly.

I remember how my daily workouts did wonders to my body when I was pregnant. I recovered quickly after my delivery. When I was pregnant, I would go for walks, do yoga, and meditate to relax my mind and my body. Although I changed my workout routine because I could not do hard exercises throughout those days, I still managed to take time out of every day for some light physical activity.

Regular cardio and HIIT workouts can counter these factors by helping you lose weight and build muscle mass. Most importantly, the workouts will also help you to burn excess calories that would otherwise accumulate as body fat. Research shows that if you keep up with a regular exercise routine, you will increase your chances of maintaining your weight loss.

According to Dr. Robyn Gmyrek, founder of Columbia University's Cosmetic Skin and Laser Center, cellulite appearance is caused by the fat cells that push up against the skin over fibrous connective tissue bands. The amount of cellulite varies from person to person according to genetics, age, and gender. Unfortunately, women are more prone to cellulite because they have higher levels of estrogen in their bodies.

Some women think that they can get rid of their cellulite and stretch marks overnight by applying some lotion to their bodies. The advertisements for these products make false promises. There is only one formula to treat your cellulite—a healthy diet, regular strength training, and cardio exercises. These exercises will help your body to build and tone your muscles, which will decrease the appearance of cellulite.

So why try all those expensive surgeries and lotions when you can benefit from an all-natural home remedy for free?

Rejuvenates Skin

Who doesn't love that natural post-workout glow? I know I do. Studies have revealed that regular cardio can revitalize your skin and protect you from different ailments like psoriasis, rosacea, acne, and pigmentation. Your aim should be to make sure that proper care is being taken toward your skin to keep it as vibrant and healthy as possible.

Doing regular cardio exercises can increase blood circulation and provide your skin with a good dose of the oxygenated blood it requires to glow. Pumping up your heart rate will nourish your skin cells as your blood carries oxygen and essential nutrients to the cells throughout your body and skin.

Another benefit of cardio is that it makes you sweat, which helps your pores completely flush out any of the oil, dirt, and bacteria from your skin which would otherwise lead to spots, blemishes, or clogged pores. However, you should always make sure to have a good scrub or a hot shower after exercising to wash away all the sweat you've accumulated from working so hard!

Hopefully, these guidelines have provided you with proper reasons for doing cardio and strength training without fail. Initially, if you don't feel like hitting the gym, start by doing some home workouts like jumping rope, weight-lifting, brisk walking, or light aerobics. Moreover, it is also important for you to understand that the excess of anything is bad, so try not to overdo any of the abovementioned exercises because it could adversely affect your body and cause injuries.

Although it's great to engage in any type of physical activity to achieve your weight loss goal, you should know that there's so much more to gain aside from a toned tummy and sculpted arms. As discussed earlier, the benefits of working out for women go way beyond the waistline.

So, try to enjoy the other advantages as well, and enjoy your workout routine to the fullest every day. Play your favorite song on your phone before you start exercising, or search for some relaxing music to accompany your meditation or yoga. Trust me, it's going to make you feel so calm and peaceful from the inside, and you will close out your practice still wanting more.

Now that you have thousands of reasons to squeeze some rocking workouts into your day, it's time to make the most energetic exercise plan for yourself and start engaging in cardio and strength training to the best of your ability.

"Yoga is the journey
of the self
through the self
to the self."

—The Bhagavad Gita

Flexibility/Balance
and Yoga

*M*ost people consider flexibility to be something in-born instead of earned. Although genetics can play an important role in determining your flexibility level, you should know that everybody has room for improvement when it comes to stretching exercises.

Since our childhood, we have been observing how many of our PE teachers focused on those sit-ups and jumping jacks but never really explained the exact benefits of flexibility. Most people don't know about the benefits of stretching. Therefore, it's harder for them to drum up the motivation to improve at it.

Contrary to what you might think, flexibility is not only about touching your toes or putting your foot behind your head. It's something much more than that.

According to The College of Sports Medicine (ACSM), "flexibility is the range of motion of a joint or group of joints per the skeletal muscles (and not any external forces)." Being flexible in all of your muscle groups helps prevent injuries, increases range of motion, improves circulation, promotes better posture, and reduces stiffness in your body.

In this section, I am going to discuss numerous ways in which you can incorporate stretching exercises into your daily routine. The American College of Sports Medicine states that a mere 10 minutes of flexibility exercises 2x/week can give you tremendous results! Personally, I like to stretch after every workout for about 10 minutes since my muscles are warm and I'm able to stretch that much better.

The researchers of ACSM talk about the two components of flexibility: static and dynamic. Static flexibility is the range of motion of an individual without movement. For instance, how far you can stretch/reach without moving. On the contrary, dynamic flexibility is the full range of motion of a given joint achieved by using your muscles and external forces exerted by yourself. For instance, lowering into a deep squat or doing arm circles is a form of dynamic flexibility.

Each one of us has a different level of flexibility. The general rule of thumb is that more flexible muscles promote greater mobility. In other words, you can say that you can't be mobile without your muscles being flexible. That's because flexible muscles make movement easier and more comfortable, as compared to stiff muscles. It allows your joints to move in proper sequence and helps you to load the right muscles and joints to perform exercises.

Mobility is an amazing tendency of the human body, making everything from HIIT class to cardio to reaching the top cabinet easier. "Improved range of motion makes the activities of daily living more feasible and enjoyable. It makes physical activity more enjoyable, it eases aches and pains, and it even improves posture," Jessica Matthews, doctor of behavioral health, explains.

However, we need to note that mobility and flexibility aren't the same thing, although we often use these terms interchangeably. Mobility is basically our joints' ability to move through its anatomically possible range of motion, which can be influenced by flexibility and other factors. Your flexibility is measured by how much your muscles and tendons around the joints can extend or lengthen with minimal effort.

Jereme Schumacher, PT, DPT, and a physical therapist at Bespoke Treatments, defines flexibility as "the ability to achieve specific joint ranges of motion in a passive manner without direct active muscle activation. Mobility, on the other hand, is when you actively move through a range of motion."

Stretching exercises are helpful in reducing the risk of injuries, stress levels, muscle tension, stiffness, and poor blood circulation. Jessica Matthews, DBH, and the author of *Stretching to Stay Young* states, "Everything from poor posture and improper body mechanics to repetitive movement patterns and sedentary behavior can limit our flexibility."

"You are only as young
as your spine is flexible."

—Joseph Pilates

Stretching Exercises
for Your Daily Workout

*H*ere is a list of some stretching exercises that will help you to enhance your muscles' flexibility and strength:

- Seated shoulder stretch
- IT band stretch
- Triceps stretch
- Butterfly stretch
- Quadriceps stretch
- Standing hamstring stretch
- Lower back stretch
- Lunge with spinal twist
- Shoulder stretch
- Upper back stretch
- Bicep stretch
- Figure four stretch
- Pigeon stretch
- Calf stretch
- Frog stretch
- Hip flexor stretch

WARNING:
Yoga has been known
to cause
health and happiness.

Yoga and Pilates

*T*he term "yoga" has been derived from the Sanskrit word "Yuji," which means yoke or union. It is an ancient practice that brings together mind and body. Yoga incorporates numerous breathing exercises, meditation, and poses designed to encourage relaxation, improve blood circulation, and reduce stress levels and anxiety.

Yoga benefits our mental and physical health at the same time and promotes a feeling of freshness within our mind and body. It is suitable for people of all ages, as it does not have any side effects when done correctly. Yoga can help you recover quickly from an illness, surgery, or a chronic condition. It also helps you to feel more energized and happier. It can literally heal your soul from depression and make you almost tension-free and more relaxed.

Many people think yoga is all about slow movements, meditating, or holding poses, but that's not necessarily true. Yoga is something more than just these things. There are also fast-moving yoga (flows) and HIIT yoga (incorporates yoga poses with high-intensity interval training-cardio). People who know me personally have a clear idea that I am not the most "zen" person, but I do love yoga for how it truly helps me to feel energized, yet relaxed.

Yoga can be for everyone! After I do my yoga, I feel like I have so much energy, and I also feel more flexible! There are so many benefits of yoga, such as increasing flexibility and muscle strength, lowering blood pressure, promoting better balance, maintaining a healthy weight, decreasing stress levels, coping with depression, and achieving mental clarity.

There are many different types of yoga you can choose from. My favorite type of yoga is the heated Vinyasa flow, which heats the room to 100°F. It really helps with my flexibility, and the heat makes it a bit more intense. You just have to find the ones that work best for you.

I am mentioning some of my favorite ones below to give you a better understanding:

- Hatha yoga (really good for beginners)
- Vinyasa flow (my personal favorite)
- Ashtanga
- Bikram
- Yin yoga
- Restorative yoga
- HIIT yoga
- Prenatal yoga
- Acro yoga
- Aerial yoga (which is also a lot of fun)
- Iyengar yoga (focuses on alignment)

Like yoga, Pilates is another form of exercise that I like to incorporate into my fitness routine. It is a low-impact exercise that strengthens muscles while improving posture alignment, balance, the core, and flexibility. You may be seeing Pilates studios popping up where you live, as it is becoming more popular with time.

Basically, there are two kinds of Pilates: mat classes or reformer classes. As the name says, the "mat class" does not involve big equipment, whereas the "reformer" Pilates includes a machine called a reformer that helps to guide you through your Pilates exercises.

I really love to incorporate yoga and Pilates into my exercise routines. I make sure to incorporate both of them into my fitness routine for about four to five days a week, along with HIIT, cardio, or strength training. Pilates helps so much with strengthening my core and elongating my muscles. I believe that doing both yoga and Pilates helps in balancing out my more intense workouts.

"In a nutshell, your health,
wealth, happiness, fitness,
and success depend on your
HABITS."

—Joanna Jast

Pilates Exercises
for Your Daily Workout

These are great examples of pilates exercises that you can utilize regularly to improve your strength and flexibility:

- Swimming
- Leg lifts
- Shoulder bridge
- Tabletop
- Alternating single leg stretch
- Toe taps
- Roll down
- The hundred
- Side leg raises
- Plank
- Arm circles
- Swan dive

Exercise is the most powerful medicine for your mental and physical health. It strengthens your cardiovascular system which allows your heart to improve blood circulation in your body. Regular workouts help to keep plaque from building up in your arteries, increase flexibility, and reduce blood pressure and chronic health issues.

Working out regularly helps you to manage a healthy weight because workouts make your tissues more sensitive to insulin, meaning that the cells throughout your body easily absorb and burn blood sugar for energy.

Out of all of these advantages to physical activity, one of my favorites is that it creates positive physiological changes in the brain that lead to an increased sense of well-being, confidence, and an improved mood.

Fitness isn't about looking good—it's about feeling unstoppable, strong, badass, and beautiful in your own skin!

"Strength does not come
from physical capacity.
It comes from an
indomitable will."

—Gandhi

What Are Core Exercises?

A strong core is one of the most valuable assets of the body. For beginners, a strong and stable midsection should be enough to provide you with better balance, help to reduce your back pain, and improve your body posture.

I cannot emphasize enough the importance of doing core exercises. Your core is the center of all of your movement. Strengthening your core helps you to not only tone your mid-section but it also promotes the balance of your entire body.

Your core is made up of several muscles, including your rectus abdominis (long muscle that runs the length of the front of the abdominal wall), transverse abdominis (the deepest internal core muscle that wraps around your sides and spine), erector spinae (your lower back muscles), and the internal and external obliques (side muscles near your abdomen).

Most of the core exercises involve working with various combinations of your muscles. Therefore, you don't have to target specific areas, like sit-ups, to challenge these muscles. Some of the best and most efficient core exercises are the ones that work on the entire muscle group all at once, which in return helps keep your muscles balanced.

According to Harvard Health Publishing, a strong core is extremely important because it acts as the main connector between your upper and lower body. Your core plays a huge role in everyday activities such as getting out of bed, walking, bending over to pick something up, and standing upright.

It is used for many of the big and small movements your body makes, including laughing. Have you ever laughed so hard that your stomach started to hurt? I can tell you—that is the best kind of laughter! The bonus is that it incorporates using your core muscles!

A strong core will assist your everyday life, reduce the risk of low back pain, promote balance and stability, and boost your confidence. The best exercise you can do for the core is a plank. I love doing planks! I like to incorporate them into my daily exercise routine. The best part is how many variations there are of it.

The most typical plank is the one in which you use your hands or elbows to hold your body up. However, a lot of other planks are also easy to incorporate, like side planks, up/down planks, shoulder tap planks, one leg planks, saw planks, and planks with hands on weights or with feet on Bosu balls.

There's so much variety to keep you fresh and energized every day you work your core!

"Work hard in silence. Let success be your noise."

—Frank Ocean

How Do Core Exercises Benefit Your Body?

*C*ore exercises should be part of your exercise routine and performed a few times each week. Not only do core exercises give you a stronger, tighter-looking core but they also help your hip, pelvis, and back work together. When they all work together, it helps you gain better balance and stability.

Some benefits of core exercises include the following:

> **Alleviate Back Pain:** Researchers state that people with weak core muscles have an increased risk of injuries, backache, and leg pain because they lack adequate spine support. Core-strengthening exercises, like yoga and Pilates, can help reduce discomfort and pain in bodies, improve mobility, and support the spine.

> **Improve Posture:** Core-strengthening exercises work wonders for people who are looking to improve their posture. These workouts focus on your torso's muscles from top to bottom, helping you to stand tall with your limbs in alignment. Improving your posture can noticeably reduce your risk of disc herniation and vertebrae degeneration as well. Moreover, it also promotes better

breathing and improves blood circulation. These balance exercises help to open your airway, which makes your inhalations and exhalations easier.

Better Athletic Performance: Core-engaging and strengthening workouts can keep runners' legs and arms from tiring quickly, which helps them to build more stamina. For example, rowers engage their cores as they paddle, and a stronger core allows them to pull comparatively harder and faster. Similarly, baseball pitchers are said to get the power for their curveballs as much from their cores as they do their arms, or you could say, maybe more. Your core is basically the connection between your upper and lower body. It allows a golfer to swing the club and strike his ball, or a tennis player to serve and optimize his racquet speed. It's essential for better athletic performance.

Improved Balance: Poor balance can be both alarming and disturbing at the same time. A few of the factors that contribute to having poor balance are lower body weakness, vestibular dysfunction, and neurological deficits. According to researchers, core-strengthening exercises can improve your body's dynamic balance if you perform them consistently.

Safer Everyday Movement: Core-strengthening activities are said to promote safer movement of the body. For example, they can help you with maintaining balance while hiking up a mountain, carrying groceries, hoisting children, and walking up a steep flight of stairs. You are also less likely to get an injury when your core is strong. Not only do you have better control of your muscles but you can more easily protect yourself and feel safe if you're ever accidentally caught off-balance.

A strong core helps you do daily activities such as tie your shoe, reach for something on a higher shelf, walk, and run. Plus it helps you reach your fitness goals. I always like to incorporate core into my daily workouts so I can try to avoid an injury. I know that the stronger my core is, my back, posture, balance, and athletic activities will all benefit.

"The difference between try and triumph is a little umph."

—Marvin Phillips

Core-Strengthening Exercises for Your Daily Workout

*T*his is a list of exercises to help strengthen your core. My personal favorite is at the top!

- Planks
- Plank shoulder taps
- Butterfly sit-up
- Dead bug
- Half-kneeling wood chop
- High-boat to low-boat
- Body saw
- Side bend
- Jackknife sit-up
- Hollow body rock
- C-curve

"She believed she could,
so she did."

—R.S. Grey

Afterword

I have this quote hanging in my girls' room and on a bracelet that my girls and I all wear. It also serves as my mantra. I like to see it as a daily reminder to continue to reach for the stars and never give up!

For a long time, it has been one of my goals to write this book, and I am so excited that you are a part of my dreams! One of my biggest goals in life is to continue to inspire women to be the best, healthiest versions of themselves.

Now that I have accomplished one of my goals, it's time for you to do the same. Just believe in yourself. I believe in you, but nothing will happen until you trust yourself and know that you are worth it! YOU GOT THIS!

I have been working in the health/fitness field for over thirty years and have seen tens of thousands of people reach their big and small goals. We have celebrated each one, big or small, because all of the small ones add up, leading you to the bigger goals!

I have worked with people who have all different types of health issues, such as obesity, diabetes, PCOS, high blood pressure, depression, heart conditions, and more. I have seen positive results from most of my clients' experiences because they have been consistent and dedicated to changing their lifestyles to become healthier and happier. Many of them end up decreasing the doses of their medications or coming off of them completely.

I want you to remember that you can take baby steps—not everyone can jump in with two feet, but each small change matters. Only you can make these changes, and it will only work when you make the changes for yourself and not for anyone else! I can guide you and give you tips and strategies, but you are the only one that can make them happen. To do it, *you need to believe in yourself.*

If you start to get off track, remind yourself why you started this health journey. Sometimes life throws us curveballs, so when this happens, go back to writing in your food journals and exercise logs, write your short-term goals for each week, and stay positive.

Remind yourself that you are stronger than you think! Sometimes it also helps to make a vision board with motivational, positive quotes and pictures of your goals and dreams. I have a vision board that I look at every day, and it helps to remind me that I can do anything I put my mind to!

For those of you who are trying to lose weight, I want you to remember something that my doctor told me after I gave birth to my son. She told me that it took nine months (well, eight for me since he was born early) to put on the weight and that I needed to give myself the same amount of time to lose it. So, if you have weight you would like to lose—*you did not gain it overnight.* Be patient with yourself, stay consistent, and it will come off.

As we discussed in previous chapters, you need to be doing this for yourself and you need to surround yourself with people who will support you, not those who will bring you down! When you have the right people supporting you, it makes a huge difference in whether you stick with your health journey or not.

Before reading this book, you may have thought that leading a healthy, positive life was hard, but now you can see that it is not. You need to make healthy choices when it comes to the food you put in your body, getting seven hours of sleep each night, incorporating different types of exercises into your workouts, keeping your stress levels low, and having a positive mindset.

Using guided meditation can really help with stress levels, as well. But I do have to confess that, often when I am stressed, I just need a good, hard workout. You can ask my family, sometimes I just say, "Ugh … I am having a bad day. I'm going to work out!"

As I share my knowledge and experiences, my goal is to inspire all women to live healthy, happy lives. We are all beautiful and blessed with different qualities and strengths, and I believe in every single one of us!

Every word in this book has been written with love, and I hope I have inspired you to change your habits into healthy ones. You can become the best version of yourself by making small changes and setting short-term goals!

I hope that you take all the strategies and tips in this book and incorporate them into your daily life. The first step is the hardest, but it is worth it. *You are worth the effort.*

Thank you for being a part of my journey, and I cannot wait to see where your path leads you!

YOU GOT THIS!

Being healthy and fit
is not a fad or a trend.
It is a lifestyle!

PART FIVE
Workbook

Identify Your "WHY?"
Worksheet

Why do you want to get healthier?

Ask yourself, *Why do I want to get healthier?* Write down whatever comes to mind. Then, ask again, *Why?* Write down your next answer. Do this over and over again until you tap into an emotional response. That's when you'll know you've found your "why."

_____

_____

_____

_____

_____

_____

_____

_____

_____

_____

_____

_____

_____

_____

"Setting goals is the first
step in turning the
invisible into the visible."

—Tony Robbins

Daily Goal-Setting Guide

Start off each week on a positive note. What is your favorite positive quote?

(Mine is: "She believed she could, so she did!")

_____

_____

_____

_____

_____

_____

_____

_____

_____

_____

_____

_____

_____

_____

_____

Weekly Goal-Setting Guide

What is your short-term goal for this week?

(Examples: *Go to the gym three times this week, add in more veggies at dinner, meditate for three minutes three times this week, get eight hours of sleep*, etc.)

_____

_____

_____

_____

_____

_____

_____

_____

_____

_____

_____

_____

_____

_____

_____

Long-Term
Goal-Setting Guide

What are your long-term goals?

(Example: *In six months, I want to be able to walk three miles without getting out of breath,* or *on my next blood test, I want my cholesterol to be within normal limits.*)

_____

_____

_____

_____

_____

_____

_____

_____

_____

_____

_____

_____

_____

_____

"If you want to be happy, be."

—Leo Tolstoy

Daily Quick Guide

Do something today that will put a smile on your face and make you feel good about yourself!

- Say HELLO to a stranger
- Call an old friend
- Go for a walk
- Go to the gym
- Drink water instead of soda
- Give someone a compliment
- Pay it forward when getting coffee/tea

What will you do/did you do today?

_____

_____

_____

_____

_____

_____

_____

_____

Give yourself permission to be happy!

"The goal is progress,
not perfection!"

—Kathy Freston

Weekly Quick Guide

What did you do this week that you did not do last week?

Here are a few things to jog your memory. Did you ...

- Make healthier food choices
- Drink more water
- Go for a walk
- Look in the mirror and say something positive to yourself
- Go to the gym
- Get more sleep
- Exercise
- Take some deep healing breaths or meditate

Add more here:

_____

_____

_____

_____

_____

STRIVE FOR GROWTH, NOT PERFECTION ...
And be proud of yourself for each step!

"You don't manifest
dreams without taking
chances."

—Stephen Richards

Don't let your fears stop you or hold you back, face them and conquer them!

What are your biggest fears? What is holding you back? What is weighing you down? Fear of failure, success, being judged, or being average? Write them below.

I faced some of my fears, got out of my comfort zone, and wrote this book!

YOU GOT THIS!

_____

_____

_____

_____

_____

_____

_____

_____

_____

_____

_____

_____

"Health is not about the
weight you lose, but
about the life you gain."

—Dr. Josh Axe

Nutrition Quick Guide

What changes can you make to your everyday diet this week?

This is a list of some great options for boosting your nutrition and leading a healthier lifestyle:

- Add more water
- Add more protein
- Eat five times throughout the day
- Make healthier carb choices, sweet potatoes, brown rice
- Eat more vegetables
- Smaller portions
- Skip dessert, or have fruit instead of cake
- Lean meat instead of the fattier choices
- Eat breakfast everyday
- Less juice and soda, switch to seltzer
- Bring lunch to work instead of buying
- Preparing food, so you can have good food to grab-n-go
- Choose healthy fats like nuts and avocados

Share yours here:

"The most important investment you can make is in yourself."

—Warren Buffet

Fitness Quick Guide

What changes have you made in your fitness routine this week?

- Go for a long walk?
- Strength training?
- Yoga?
- Swim?
- Jog/run?
- Do a High Intensity Interval Training (HIIT) workout?
- Park your car at the far end of the parking lot?
- Take steps instead of the elevator?
- Find a workout buddy?
- Go to the gym?

Share yours here:

_____

_____

_____

_____

_____

_____

_____

"Sleep is the golden chain
that ties health and our
bodies together."

—Thomas Dekker

Healthy Sleep Quick Guide

- Avoid napping
- Go to bed at the same time each day
- Get up at the same time each day
- Get off phone/computer one hour before bed
- Don't work in bed
- Relax your mind
- Take a hot shower/bath before bed
- Avoid eating meals before bed
- Listen to relaxing music
- No caffeine in the afternoon/evening
- Make your room dark, quiet, and comfortable
- Get some sunshine

Share yours here:

_____

_____

_____

_____

_____

_____

_____

Workout Planner

Make one for each day of the week.

MONDAY

Activity:	Duration/Distance:
Cardio	
Strength	

Grocery List Planner

Fruits:	Vegetables:
Whole Grains:	**Proteins:**

"The day she let go of the things that were weighing her down was the day she began to shine the brightest."

—Katrina Mayer

Stress Release Checklist

- Listen to music
- Take deep breaths
- Meditate
- Stretch
- Yoga
- Hot cup of herbal tea
- Cuddle with a pet
- Get some sunshine
- Exercise

And above all ...
LAUGH!

"No one is born a great cook, one learns by doing."

—Julia Child

Recipes

I have included some of my family's favorite recipes for you to try. I have also added a recipe alternative list that I believe will be very helpful. Remember to always season your food and make it very flavorful. This way you won't get bored with what you're eating. Healthy food can be delicious and savory!

CITRUS AND HERB CHICKEN

Ingredients:

- 2 tsp lemon rind, finely grated
- 3 tbsp lemon juice
- 1 tbsp Dijon mustard
- 1 tbsp fresh tarragon, chopped
- 2 tbsp fresh chives, chopped
- 2 tsp extra virgin olive oil
- 8 pieces of chicken strips
- 2 bunches of asparagus, trimmed
- 1 can cannellini beans, rinsed and drained
- 1 cup cherry tomatoes, halved
- 2 celery stalks, finely chopped

- 1 bag of baby spinach leaves
- 1 tsp Dijon mustard, set aside
- Lemon wedges, to serve

Directions:

1. Combine the lemon rind and juice, mustard, tarragon, 1 tbsp chives, and 1 tsp olive oil in a shallow glass or ceramic dish. Add the chicken and turn to coat. Cover. Place in the fridge for 30 minutes to marinate.

2. Preheat barbecue grill on medium-high, grill the chicken, and cook through. Spray the asparagus lightly with oil and grill for 1–2 minutes on each side or until lightly charred.

3. Add cannellini beans, tomato, celery, spinach, and remaining chives in a separate bowl. Combine the extra lemon juice, extra mustard, and remaining olive oil in a bowl.

4. Add the asparagus and lemon dressing to the cannellini bean mixture and gently toss to combine. Serve with lemon wedges and enjoy!

CHIA SEED PUDDING

We make this all of the time and my kids love it!

Ingredients:

- 2 tbsp chia seeds
- ½ cup of almond milk
- 1 tsp honey

- Your choice of fruit—cut-up strawberries, blueberries, raspberries

Directions: Pour ingredients into a mason jar and mix well. Cover and refrigerate for 3–4 hours. Top with your favorite fruit(s).

BERRY PROTEIN SHAKE

We like to use frozen fruit to make the shake thicker.

Ingredients:

- ¾ cup almond milk
- ½ ripe banana
- ½ cup frozen raspberries
- ½ cup frozen blueberries
- 1 scoop vanilla whey or vegan protein powder

Directions: Mix in a blender, pour into a glass, and enjoy!

SLOW COOKER BEAN STEW

I love this meal on a busy or rainy day when I don't have time to cook.

Ingredients:

- 3 cups of chicken broth
- 2 carrots, peeled & chopped
- 1 can (15 ounce) chickpeas
- 2 cans (14 ounce) fire-roasted tomatoes

- 1 red onion (chopped)
- 1 can (15 ounce) kidney beans
- 1 bunch of kale, chopped
- 2 garlic cloves, minced
- 1 tsp dried oregano
- ¼ tsp ground pepper
- 1 tbsp lemon juice
- 2 tbsp extra virgin olive oil
- 2 tbsp fresh basil leaves, chopped

Combine all of the ingredients together in your slow cooker and cover. (I always use the liner bag, for easy clean-up.) Set the slow cooker to cook on low for 6 hours. ENJOY!!

GRILLED CHICKEN LETTUCE WRAPS

Another quick and easy favorite in my house. Many times I use leftover chicken or ready-made rotisserie chicken.

Ingredients:

- 3 boneless skinless chicken breasts, either grilled or rotisserie
- Large romaine leaves or butterhead lettuce (to be used like a wrap)
- 1/2 red onion, thinly sliced
- 1 carrot, shredded
- 1 tbsp freshly-chopped cilantro
- Sliced avocado

- Sliced cucumbers
- Chili sauce or any dressing of your choice

Directions:

1. Cook chicken in a pan for 8–10 minutes on each side, or until fully cooked. (Or use ready-made rotisserie chicken.)
2. Let cool for 5 minutes, cut into strips.
3. Add meat onto lettuce
4. Add chopped veggies, avocado, cilantro, etc.
5. Add a sauce of your choice and ENJOY!

CAULIFLOWER BUFFALO WINGS

Ingredients:

- 1 head of cauliflower, cut into small pieces
- ½ cup of almond flour
- ¼ tsp pepper
- ½ tsp salt
- ¼ tsp paprika
- ½ tsp onion powder
- ¼ tsp garlic powder
- ⅛ tsp cumin
- ⅓ cup unsweetened almond milk
- ¼ cup of water
- ¼ cup buffalo sauce or hot sauce

Directions: Combine all ingredients together in a bowl (except cauliflower). Toss well with cauliflower and bake at 450°F for 25 minutes.

PROTEIN PANCAKES

Ingredients:

- 2 scoops of protein powder
- ⅓ cup for liquid egg whites
- 1 tsp baking powder
- ¼ tsp cinnamon
- 1 tbsp almond milk

Directions: Add ingredients together, scoop onto a pan, and cook over medium heat. Cook thoroughly and ENJOY!

THREE-INGREDIENT COOKIES

Ingredients:

- 3 bananas, mashed
- 2 cups of oats
- ½ cup of all-natural peanut butter
- dark chocolate chips (optional)

Directions:

1. Mix all ingredients together.
2. Form into balls.
3. Place on cookie sheets.
4. Bake at 350°F for 10–12 minutes.

ENJOY!

SALMON

This is so easy, yet very delicious!

Ingredients:

- 3–6 ounces of salmon
- 1 tbsp olive oil
- 2 garlic cloves, minced
- 1 lemon, zest only
- 1½ tbsp freshly-minced parsley
- 1 tbsp fresh dill
- salt
- black pepper

Directions:

1. Mix olive oil, garlic, lemon zest, parsley, and dill in a bowl.
2. Spread sauce over salmon.
3. Add salt and pepper.
4. Bake at 425°F for 18–20 minutes or BBQ (which I love to do & is easy to clean up).

ENJOY!

BAKED OAT BARS

Ingredients:

- 1 cup rolled oats
- ¾ cup almond milk

- 1 banana
- 1 egg
- 1 tsp baking powder
- 1 tsp cinnamon
- 1 tsp vanilla extract
- 2 tbsp honey
- Optional—dark chocolate chips, nuts, or berries

Directions:

1. Mix all ingredients. (You can add your optional ingredients to this mixture or leave them out and sprinkle on top.)
2. Pour into a nonstick baking pan (or spray the pan with nonstick cooking spray).
3. Top with dark chocolate chips, berries, or nuts! (If you chose to put these into your mixture, skip this step.)
4. Bake at 375°F for 30 minutes.
5. Let cool and cut into bars.
6. ENJOY!

CHICKEN MEATBALLS

Ingredients:

- 1 pound ground chicken or turkey
- 1 egg
- ½ cup panko Italian seasoned breadcrumbs
- ½ tsp garlic powder

- ½ tsp onion powder
- ½ tsp salt
- black pepper to taste

Directions:

1. Mix all ingredients together.
2. Roll mixture into several small balls.
3. Bake at 400°F for 25–30 minutes.

Serve with brown rice pasta, spaghetti squash, or hearts of palm pasta.

VANILLA BEAN FRAPPUCCINO

Ingredients:

- 1 cup of ice
- ½ cup cold-brewed coffee
- 1 cup almond milk
- 1 tsp vanilla extract

Directions: Blend, top with coconut whipped cream, and enjoy!

PROTEIN CHOCOLATE ICE CREAM

Ingredients:

- 1 scoop of chocolate protein powder (whey or vegan)
- 1½ cups of frozen banana
- ⅓ cup of almond milk

Directions: Blend and enjoy!

COFFEE SMOOTHIE

- 1 frozen banana
- ½ cup cold brew coffee
- 1 scoop chocolate or vanilla protein powder (whey or vegan)
- ½ cup almond milk
- 1 tbsp cocoa powder

Directions: Put all ingredients in a blender and mix. Yum!

Recipe Alternatives

Bored of your water?

Here are some options to add flavor ...

- Lemon
- Strawberries
- Cucumber and mint (my favorite)
- Raspberry lime
- Strawberry lemon
- Raspberry cucumber mint
- Oranges

Looking for some healthier pasta alternatives? Try ...

- Chickpea pasta
- Zoodles (Zucchini cut like pasta)
- Quinoa pasta
- Rice
- Hearts of palm pasta
- Red lentil pasta
- Spaghetti squash

"If you don't risk
anything, you risk even
more."

—Erica Jong

Recipe Substitution Ideas

If your recipe calls for...	Substitute with...
Sugar	Unsweetened Applesauce
Whole Milk	Skim or Low-fat Cow's Milk, Almond, Cashew, Oat Milk
Eggs	2 Egg Whites = 1 Egg or ¼ Cup of Liquid Eggs
White Flour	Almond Flour
Peanut Butter	All-Natural Peanut Butter
Heavy Cream	Evaporated Skim Milk, Low-fat Yogurt, or Nonfat Yogurt
Breadcrumbs	Panko Crumbs
Mayonnaise	Mashed Avocado or Reduced-fat Mayo
Chocolate Chips	Dark Chocolate Chips
Soy Sauce	Reduced-sodium Soy Sauce
Sautéed in Oil	Sauté in Broth

Baking Chocolate	Unsweetened Cocoa Powder
Oil-Based Marinade/ Dressing	Balsamic Vinegar, Flavored Vinegars
	Low-Sodium Broth, Herb Seasonings
Tortillas/Wraps	Lettuce
Cheese	Nutritional Yeast
White Potatoes	Sweet Potatoes
White Rice	Brown Rice, Cauliflower Rice, Quinoa

"Gratitude is the fairest
blossom which springs
from the soul."

—Henry Ward Beecher

Acknowledgments

I would like to thank my family, friends, and my publishing team for helping me turn this book into a reality.

I could not have done this without your support.

Thank you.

References

1. American College Of Sports Medicine. "Chapter 5." Essay. In *ACSMS Resources for the Exercise Physiologist.* Lippincott Williams And Wilkin, 2017.

2. Zelman, Kathleen M. "4 Steps to a Healthy Lifestyle." WebMD. Accessed February 11, 2022. https://www.webmd.com/diet/features/4-steps-healthy-lifestyle.

3. Risher, B. "5 Benefits of Flexibility and Why Flexibility Is so Important." LIVESTRONG.COM. Leaf Group. Accessed February 11, 2022. https://www.livestrong.com/article/332519-what-are-the-benefits-of-good-flexibility/.

4. "January 2012 References and Further Reading." Harvard Health, January 1, 2012. https://www.health.harvard.edu/heart-health/january-2012-references-and-further-reading.

5. Youdim, Adrienne. "Carbohydrates, Proteins, and Fats—Disorders of Nutrition." MSD Manual Consumer Version. MSD Manuals, February 7, 2022. https://www.msdmanuals.com/en-au/home/disorders-of-nutrition/overview-of-nutrition/carbohydrates,-proteins,-and-fats?query=carbohydrates%2C+proteins%2C+and+fats.

6. Bhandari, Smitha, medical reviewer. "The Effects of Stress on Your Body." WebMD. WebMD, December 8, 2017. https://www.webmd.com/balance/stress-management/effects-of-stress-on-your-body.

7. Magee, Elaine. "11 Simple Steps to a Healthy Diet." WebMD. WebMD, April 2009. https://www.webmd.com/diet/features/11-simple-steps-to-a-healthier-diet.

8. Anon. n.d. "Getting Active to Control High Blood Pressure." www.heart.org. Accessed February 12, 2022. https://www.heart.org/en/health-topics/high-blood-pressure/changes-you-can-make-to-manage-high-blood-pressure/getting-active-to-control-high-blood-pressure.

9. Projects, Contributors to Wikimedia. "Healthy Diet." Wikipedia. Wikimedia Foundation, Inc., February 4, 2022. https://en.wikidark.org/wiki/Healthy_diet.

10. Anon. n.d. "American Heart Association Recommendations for Physical Activity in Adults and Kids | American Heart Association." Retrieved from (https://www.heart.org/en/healthy-living/fitness/fitness-basics/aha-recs-for-physical-activity-in-adults).

11. Könen, Tanja, Judith Dirk, and Florian Schmiedek. "Cognitive Benefits of Last Night's Sleep: Daily Variations in Children's Sleep Behavior Are Related to Working Memory Fluctuations." Journal of Child Psychology and Psychiatry, and Allied Disciplines. U.S. National Library of Medicine, February 2015. https://www.ncbi.nlm.nih.gov/pubmed/25052368/%EF%BB%BF.

12. "Are You Getting Enough Sleep?" Centers for Disease Control and Prevention, April 21, 2021. https://www.cdc.gov/sleep/features/getting-enough-sleep.html.

About the Author

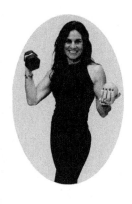

Beth Linder-Moss is a certified Health and Wellness Coach, Personal and Group Fitness Trainer, and Exercise Physiologist. She earned her Bachelor of Science degree in Exercise and Sports Science from The Pennsylvania State University. During her freshman year, she was inspired to make a career change when she received her first Group Fitness Certification.

Since that time, Beth has acquired several certifications. She is currently certified as an exercise physiologist and personal trainer through The American College of Sports Medicine, a Certified Specialist in Sports Nutrition, and a Health and Wellness Coach. In addition to her certifications, Beth possesses several supplementary exercise and nutrition-related credentials.

Beth did not stop there! She went on to create two fitness/nutrition certifications on behalf of a large national franchise and is also the author of a certification program that teaches how to incorporate High-Intensity Interval Training (HIIT) into yoga classes for a large yoga franchise.

To find out more, visit:

bethlinder-moss.com
instagram.com/beth_linder_moss
tiktok.com/@bethmoss2

Printed in Great Britain
by Amazon

40882329R00126